THETA HEALING
DIGGING FOR BELIEFS

THETA HEALING

DIGGING FOR BELIEFS

VIANNA STIBAL

HAY HOUSE

Carlsbad, California • New York City
London • Sydney • New Delhi

Published in the United Kingdom by:
Hay House UK Ltd, The Sixth Floor, Watson House,
54 Baker Street, London W1U 7BU
Tel: +44 (0)20 3927 7290; Fax: +44 (0)20 3927 7291; www.hayhouse.co.uk

Published in the United States of America by:
Hay House Inc., PO Box 5100, Carlsbad, CA 92018-5100
Tel: (1) 760 431 7695 or (800) 654 5126
Fax: (1) 760 431 6948 or (800) 650 5115; www.hayhouse.com

Published in Australia by:
Hay House Australia Ltd, 18/36 Ralph St, Alexandria NSW 2015
Tel: (61) 2 9669 4299; Fax: (61) 2 9669 4144; www.hayhouse.com.au

Published in India by:
Hay House Publishers India, Muskaan Complex, Plot No.3, B-2,
Vasant Kunj, New Delhi 110 070
Tel: (91) 11 4176 1620; Fax: (91) 11 4176 1630; www.hayhouse.co.in

A catalogue record for this book is available from the British Library.

Tradepaper ISBN: 978-1-78817-346-9
E-book ISBN: 978-1-78817-349-0

15 14 13 12 11 10 9 8 7

Interior images: 123rf/sumkinn

Printed in the United States of America

This product uses papers sourced from responsibly managed forests. For more information, see www.hayhouse.com.

CONTENTS

See the glossary for terms given in **bold**.

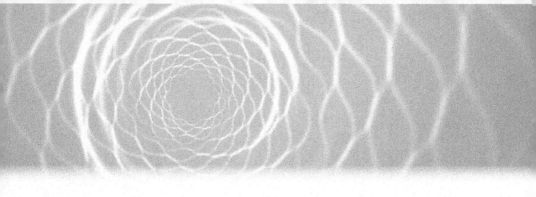

LIST OF EXERCISES

PREFACE

ThetaHealing is a philosophy and complete **healing system**, which can be used to change self-limiting beliefs and improve positive beliefs, as well as for self-understanding and evolving spiritually for the benefit of humankind.

This book is designed as an in-depth guide to digging for beliefs, and is a companion to *ThetaHealing*, *Advanced ThetaHealing*, *ThetaHealing Diseases and Disorders*, and *The Planes of Existence*.

In the first book, *ThetaHealing*, I explain the step-by-step processes of ThetaHealing reading, healing, **belief work**, **feeling work**, **digging work** and **gene work**, and offer an introduction to the **planes of existence**, as well as additional knowledge for the beginner.

The next book, *Advanced ThetaHealing*, provides a more in-depth guide to belief and feeling work, and digging, as well as deeper insights into the planes of existence and the beliefs, which I believe are essential for spiritual evolution. *Advanced ThetaHealing* expands on the first book, *ThetaHealing*, while *The Planes of Existence* defines the philosophy of ThetaHealing.

It is necessary to reach an understanding of the processes that are given in *ThetaHealing* to utilize fully the digging for beliefs practices described in this book. However, you will find a description of the ThetaHealing processes in Chapters 1–2 and the glossary – all of which you may find useful if you are new to ThetaHealing.

The energy-healing techniques used in this book are fully explained in *ThetaHealing* and *Advanced ThetaHealing*, together with the meditation practices using the **Theta brainwave**, which I believe create physical, psychological, and spiritual healing. While in a pure and divine **Theta state** of mind, we are able to connect with the **Creator of All That Is** through focused prayer. The Creator has given us the fascinating knowledge you are about to receive; it has changed my life and the lives of many others.

There is, however, one requirement that is absolute with ThetaHealing and the techniques described in this book: you must have a central belief in an energy that flows through all things. Some might call this the 'Creator of All That Is,' 'Creator,' or 'God.' With study and practice anyone can do it; anyone who believes in God or the All That Is essence that flows through all things. ThetaHealing has no religious affiliation. Neither are its processes specific to any age, sex, race, color, creed, or religion. Anyone with a pure belief in God or the creative force can access and use the branches of the ThetaHealing tree, and I realize that the Creator has many different names: God, the Life Force, Allah, Creator of All That Is, Goddess, Jesus, Holy Spirit, Source, and Yahweh.

Even though I am sharing this information with you, I don't accept any responsibility for the changes that may occur from its use. The responsibility is yours, a responsibility you assume when you realize that you have the power to change your life, as well as the lives of others.

NOTE TO THE
READER

After teaching ThetaHealing classes for many years, I began to see irregularities in how some students were digging for the bottom or key belief in a session.

Some students may have developed bad habits due to being taught by early ThetaHealing teachers, who had learned (or created) the wrong way to dig, while other students were not taught any of the digging practices. Some students downloaded negative beliefs, or only downloaded long lists in belief-work sessions, while others did belief work but didn't use downloads. Some practitioners were doing good belief work, but it wasn't as effective as it could be, and their clients needed more sessions than was necessary to heal. Some students didn't read the digging explanations in the basic and advanced books.

Digging is one of the most important features of ThetaHealing but every year students came to my teacher's class with bad habits. The digging class was designed to help them dig effectively and quickly for beliefs, and this book is the result.

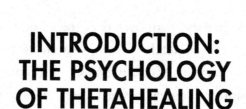

INTRODUCTION: THE PSYCHOLOGY OF THETAHEALING

There have been volumes written on beliefs, emotions, and emotional states; and many theories about how they are created – most of which attempt to explain *how* they work within psychology, physiology, philosophy, neurology, sociology, endocrinology, and psychotherapy. The question they all ask is, 'How do we define a feeling, belief, or emotion? Where and how does it exist in the brain and what is it?'

In modern science, many of the concepts about emotions and beliefs are, in essence, learning processes of theoretical speculation, with one idea building on the other. To some psychologists, a feeling is a subjective experience which is the result of an emotional state. We can view the result of an emotional state through verbal and physical reactions, but we can't *mechanistically see* how they are formed – except by taking an electroencephalography reading to monitor brainwaves and, more recently, a CT scan. We can, however, surmise that emotions are sent through the body by way of chemical and electrical messages via the body's circulatory and neurological systems.

Some psychologists propose that our emotional states are essentially biologically driven responses to social and environmental factors. According to these theories, there are six basic emotions: anger, disgust, fear, happiness, sadness, and surprise. These basic emotions then blend to form more complex emotions. A good example of this would be feeling anger and disgust at the same time, and these emotions blend to form the feeling of contempt. (Please understand that these concepts are at least, in part, theories about emotions.)

None of this, however, explains *why* we develop a particular belief, or one has been sent down to us. Is a belief an emotional state? Where is it in the brain? How is it formed? Why does one person develop certain beliefs and not another?

One thing seems certain: beliefs are mental objects that are deeply embedded in the brain and like memories can solidify into positive or negative states. Therefore, the next question is, how do we recognize our beliefs and how can they be changed if needed? Hatred, prejudice, and discrimination are but a few examples of negative beliefs that can solidify into something beyond an emotion, although they are also a source of negative emotions, whereas beliefs about prayer, meditation, love, goodwill, and so on have a tendency to create positive emotions and feelings. Some scientists speculate that beliefs solidify in the same way that memories form in the brain, but once solidified, how do you change them?

Kathleen Taylor, a neuroscientist at Oxford University says, 'If you challenge them [beliefs]… then they are going to weaken slightly. If that is combined with very strong reinforcement of new beliefs, then you're going to get a shift in emphasis from one to the other.'[1]

BELIEFS – A PORTAL TO THE SUBCONSCIOUS

Belief and **digging work** are an essential part of ThetaHealing and can be easily understood from a psychological viewpoint as a way of directly opening a portal into the **subconscious** mind in order to create change. Observing people in belief-work sessions indicates that there is a bubble of protection around the ocean of the subconscious – at least in some people. This field of protection is created in a natural process so the hard drive of the subconscious can insulate us from pain – or what it perceives might be painful to us – should we attempt to change the beliefs (or **programs**) that have formed over our lifetime.

The brain works like a biological super-computer, assessing information and responding. How we respond to an experience depends on the information given to the subconscious, and how it is received and interpreted. When a belief has been accepted as 'real' by the mind, it becomes crystallized as a program and placed into the hard drive of the subconscious. As in computing, ThetaHealing calls beliefs 'programs' because the hard drive of the subconscious 'acts out' these beliefs, regardless of whether they are negative or positive.

A program can be for our benefit or become a detriment, depending on what it is and how we react to it. For example, living with the hidden program of 'I can't succeed' may result in losing everything, even after years of success, or in self-defeating behaviors; and because the program is unconscious it continues to be self-sabotaging. These types of programs, which likely formed in childhood, lie deep in the subconscious mind, waiting for the opportunity to be reasserted into reality.

This is also why, as we learn and grow over our lifetime, many of us find that change and growth are not our friends. When we are children, experiences teach us change can be painful, even dangerous. Trauma experienced in childhood – perhaps due to changing schools, divorce, death, or some other reason – causes a bubble of protection to form around the subconscious, as a way of insulating us from pain. As we grow older, change and growth (as they are perceived by the Western mindset) are also perceived as being painful. Events such as losing or changing jobs, relationship break-ups, or our bodies aging, can also mean our perception of change becomes progressively more negative. As the subconscious internalizes these learned behaviors – some of which may not be to our benefit – it knows that there are monsters in the deep, and some of these behaviors could be painful if they were contacted directly and an attempt made for positive change – and so the bubble of protection stays in place. The older we become, the more and more difficult it becomes to make changes that might be painful for us, and so the layers of protection become thicker and thicker. Belief work is a way of piercing through the layers of the bubble to the subconscious mind and making change without creating pain.

Belief work empowers us with the ability to remove and replace any negative programs with positive, beneficial ones through the perception that change can be created through the most powerful force in the universe, the energy of subatomic particles. How this essence is perceived is up to the individual. Some people might call this essence 'God,' but others might perceive it scientifically. Either way it gives a focal point for creating tangible change in our lives. In this process a belief, which is both external yet internal, is accepted as more powerful than any other in our minds.

THE PROCESS OF CREATING CHANGE

Using **energy testing** (see Chapter 2), we can perceive what belief programs are held in the subconscious and at which of **the four levels of belief (core, genetic, history, and soul)** – which we believe are inherent within us. Energy testing is a direct procedure – via a reaction to stimuli – to test for your own or a client's energy field, or All That Is essence, and an accurate way of revealing whether a belief program exists and bringing it into **conscious** awareness. The belief program can then be released and a new one downloaded in its place. In other words, the client *believes* the belief program has been released and there is a new one in its place.

Energy testing is helpful for those just starting to use belief work and for those clients who need 'proof' that something is happening. However, once you become more familiar with the synchronistic interaction of digging for the bottom or key belief (which we will explore in more detail in later chapters), you won't have to use the rather mechanistic process of energy testing for every belief, as the client will begin to make intuitive quantum leaps in the interaction process.

Most important is that the energy-testing tool teaches us that we can access the subconscious without pain and make changes within it. When enough of these programs are altered, the mind learns that it doesn't need to protect us and, eventually, we are given direct access to our subconscious. At this point, we can begin to spontaneously make changes without energy testing. Any further changes that are needed begin to come to us in dreams in our subconscious and then openly to our conscious mind, as we go about our day-to-day lives. We find that while change might still be difficult, it is no longer so overwhelming that we are afraid of it. At this point, we are automatically doing belief work on ourselves, instantaneously creating change within ourselves that then manifests and extends to the more material aspects of our lives.

However, in order to change beliefs, the subconscious must feel comfortable about releasing them. The four levels of belief are a way of opening the doors to the subconscious and creating change to programs that might otherwise stay in place. This is because once the subconscious accepts the idea of the four belief levels, it has a structure within which to manifest change and growth.

The feeling work is a suggestion to the subconscious mind that there may be feelings that it hasn't experienced or rejected for some reason in the past. It is also suggested that these feelings can be downloaded from the Divine and because this suggestion comes from a divine place, the subconscious is more likely to accept the **feeling download** presented to it and permit the subconscious to accept positive change.

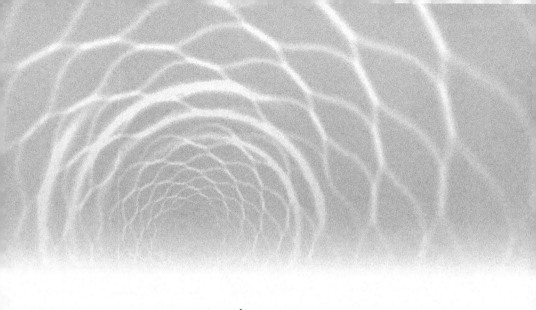

Chapter 1

THE
THETA
TECHNIQUE

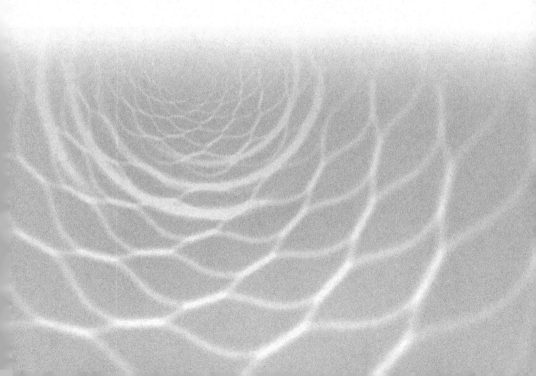

As I described in the Introduction, belief work is important in bringing any belief programs, which are preventing us from healing or moving forward, into our conscious awareness. When digging for beliefs, you will be utilizing a technique that takes you to a Theta brainwave and, if you are new to ThetaHealing, you may find this chapter useful in getting an overview of the branches of the Theta technique.

The basic healing and **reading** techniques of ThetaHealing are really quite easy to follow. However, *the modus operandi* of these procedures is visualization, which may not come naturally to you so it's a good idea to practice the techniques given in this chapter before starting any belief work. What we have found, however, is that everyone can learn to visualize and, if you follow the instructions at your own pace, you will become skilled at it.

THE THETAHEALING TREE

Healings and readings are based upon the power of a connection to the Creator and focused thought. In order to have this connection and focus your thoughts, you must first recognize your intuitive abilities. Then, in order to understand the process, learn all you can about your inherent potential.

The following terms refer to the first 'branches' of the ThetaHealing 'tree' we use to 'go up and seek God':

- The power of words and thought

- Brainwaves

- Psychic senses and chakras

- Free agency; co-creation

- The command or request (the command is to your subconscious, the request is to the Creator)

- The power of observation-visualization and being the witness

- The Creator of All That Is of the **Seventh Plane of Existence**

THETA STATE OF MIND

The next part of the process is to understand how to utilize the **Theta state** of mind in readiness for belief work. There are five different brainwaves: beta, alpha, theta, delta, and gamma. These brainwaves are constantly in motion as the brain is consistently producing waves in all five frequencies. Everything that we do and say is regulated by the frequency of our brainwaves.

A **Theta brainwave state** is a very deep state of relaxation; a dream state, which is always creative, inspirational, and characterized by spiritual sensations. We believe this state allows us to access the subconscious mind and opens a direct conduit of communication to the divine.

I believe when we practice meditation and say the word 'God,' we are able to hold a conscious Theta brainwave. In this conscious Theta state of mind, I believe we can create anything, change our reality instantly, and send our consciousness beyond this mortal body to connect to the Seventh Plane of Existence 'All That Is' energy, which is inherent in all things throughout the universe. Many studies[2] have shown that the healer, and the person being healed, drop into a Theta-Delta frequency, and this may explain the visionary experiences of some healers.

So, before starting to dig for beliefs – whether for yourself or with a client – use the following All That Is energy meditation to go the Seventh Plane of Existence; it will unlock doors in your mind and connect you with the purest essence of the All That Is energy. This mental road map will stimulate the neurons in your brain and connect you to the energy of creation.

ROAD MAP TO ALL THAT IS MEDITATION (EXTENDED VERSION)

In this meditation, which is an extended version of the one given in *Planes of Existence*, you go on a journey to find the Creator-self inside you – who is of the highest intelligence and perfect love – and travel outward to the cosmic consciousness at the same time.

1. Begin by sending your consciousness down into the center of Mother Earth, into the energy of All That Is.

2. Now bring the energy of All That Is up through your feet and into your body.

3. Now bring the energy up through all your seven chakras, then up and out through the top of your head. Imagine this energy as a beautiful ball of light and see yourself within it. Take some time to notice what color it is.

4. Project your consciousness out past the stars and imagine going up above the universe.

5. Imagine going into the light above the universe; it is a big, beautiful light. Imagine going up through that light, and you will see another bright light, and another, and another. There are many bright lights, so keep going.

6. Between the lights, there is a little bit of dark light, but this is just a layer before the next light, so keep going.

7. Finally, there is a great big, bright golden light. Go through it. When you go through it, you will see an energy that is darker at first – a thick watery, jelly-like substance that is made up of all the colors of the rainbow. When you go into this jelly-like substance, you see that it changes colors – this is where the Laws reside and here you will see all kinds of shapes and colors. In the distance, there is a white iridescent light; it is a white-blue color, like a pearl. Head toward that light. Avoid the deep blue light because this is the Law of Magnetism. It is possible to become entranced in the essence of the Laws, so be sure to go to the next light.

8. As you get closer to the white iridescent light, you will see a mist of a pink color. This is the Law of Compassion and it will guide you into the special place of the Seventh Plane of Existence. You may see that the pearlescent light is the shape of a rectangle, like a window; it is the opening to the Seventh Plane.

9. Now go through the opening. Go deep within it. You will be in a white light that sparkles. At first this light may have a few sparkles of pearlescent blue and pink within it, but it is mostly a luminescent snow-white light. Feel it go through your body. It feels light, but it has essence. You can feel it going through you; it is as if you can no longer feel the separation between your own body and the energy. You become the Creator of All That Is, of the highest intelligence and greatest love. Don't worry, your body will not disappear but become perfect and healthy. Remember there is just energy here, not people or things, so if you see people, go higher. It is from this place, that the 'Creator of All That Is' can perform healings that will heal instantly and that you can create all aspects of your life.

Once you have an understanding of this meditation and have become familiar with its practice, you are ready to use the reading and healing processes, given below, to release, replace, and dig for beliefs. Both the following descriptions of the reading and healing are shortened versions from *ThetaHealing*.

READING

The process of the reading is a means for a healer to send their consciousness into another person's space to do a body scan. The reading is simple:

1. Center yourself.

2. Begin by sending your consciousness down into the center of Mother Earth, into the energy of All That Is.

3. Bring the energy up through your feet, into your body, and bring the energy up through all the chakras.

4. Go up through your crown chakra, raise and project your consciousness out past the stars to the universe.

5. Go beyond the universe, through layers of light, through a golden light, past the jelly-like substance, which are the Laws, into a pearly, iridescent white light to the Seventh Plane of Existence.

6. Make the command or request, 'Creator of All That Is, it is commanded or requested to witness the reading in [insert the name of the person]. Thank you! It is done. It is done. It is done.'

7. Go into the client's space.

8. Imagine going into their body to turn on a light.

9. If any part of their body doesn't light up as you are going through it, there may be a problem in that area.

10. Once finished, rinse yourself off with the Seventh Plane of Existence energy and stay connected to it.

The next step in the reading is the healing.

HEALING

The 'Creator of All That Is' is the healer and you are just the observer witnessing it. The healing is simple:

1. Center yourself.

2. Begin by sending your consciousness down into the center of Mother Earth, into the energy of All That Is.

3. Bring the energy up through your feet, into your body, and bring the energy up through all the chakras.

4. Go up through your crown chakra, raise and project your consciousness out past the stars to the universe.

5. Go beyond the universe, through layers of light, through a golden light, past the jelly-like substance, which are the Laws, into a pearly, iridescent white light to the Seventh Plane of Existence.

6. Make the command or request, 'Creator of All That Is, it is commanded or requested to witness a healing in [*insert the name of the person*]. Thank you! It is done. It is done. It is done.'

7. Go into the person's space and witness the Creator heal the person.

8. Stay in the challenged area until the healing energy is finished.

9. Once finished, rinse yourself off with the Seventh Plane of Existence energy and stay connected to it.

In order for a healing to happen, the recipient must want to restore themselves to health and the healer must *believe* it is possible. If the person doesn't want to be healed, or doesn't think they can be healed, the healing technique can be used in a different way to change beliefs.

—

**Belief work empowers us with the ability
to remove and replace negative programs
with positive, beneficial programs
from the Creator of All That Is.**

—

BELIEF WORK

Belief work is at the heart of ThetaHealing and is a means of changing limiting beliefs that have become programs in the subconscious before digging for the bottom or key belief.

Programs and belief levels

When a belief has been accepted as 'real' by the body, mind, or soul it becomes a program. These programs can be for our benefit or detriment – depending on what they are and how we react to them. ThetaHealing teaches that there are four levels on which belief programs are held (core, genetic, history, and soul), which you can use as a guide for removing and replacing programs in your belief-work sessions.

Core beliefs

Core beliefs are what we are taught in this life and have accepted from childhood. These beliefs have become part of us and are held as energy in the frontal lobe of the brain.

Genetic beliefs

In this level, beliefs are inherited from our ancestors or are being added to the genes in this life. These beliefs are energies stored in the morphogenetic field around our physical DNA. This field of knowledge is what tells the mechanics of the DNA what to do.

History beliefs

This level concerns memories from past lives, deep genetic memories, or collective-consciousness experiences that we carry into the present. These memories are held in our auric field.

Soul beliefs

This level is all that a person 'is.' These are the deepest and most pervading of all the belief programs and are pulled off the completeness of the individual, beginning at the heart chakra, outward.

Use these four levels of belief as your guide for removing and replacing programs in your belief-work sessions.

As described in Chapter 1, we can use energy testing to find belief programs on all four levels of belief (see Chapter 2 for the correct energy-testing methods and processes). Energy testing is a direct procedure that you can use to test for a 'Yes' or 'No' response to ascertain whether a certain belief is present.

PROCESS TO CHANGE A BELIEF

The following process is an example only. The complete process of releasing beliefs from the four levels is given in *ThetaHealing*.

1. Center yourself.

2. Begin by sending your consciousness down into the center of Mother Earth, into the energy of All That Is.

3. Bring the energy up through your feet, into your body, and through all the chakras.

4. Go up through your crown chakra, raise and project your consciousness out past the stars to the universe.

5. Go beyond the universe, through layers of light, through a golden light, past the jelly-like substance, which are the Laws, into a pearly, iridescent white light to the Seventh Plane of Existence.

6. Make the command or request, 'Creator of All That Is, it is commanded or requested that the program belief of [*whatever the belief is*] be pulled on all four levels, cancelled, resolved on the history level, and sent to God's light from [*say the person's name*], replaced with [*whatever God tells you*]. Thank you! It is done. It is done. It is done.'

7. Witness the program and energy associated with [*whatever the belief is*] being pulled, cancelled, resolved on the history level, sent to God's light and replaced with the new program of [*whatever God tells you*] from the Creator.

8. Once finished, rinse yourself off with the Seventh Plane of Existence energy and stay connected to it.

DIGGING

Digging is energy testing for the key belief that has all the other beliefs stacked on top of it. In a one-on-one session, the practitioner is the investigator and energy tests the client's statements to find clues to their key belief.

You might find it helpful to visualize the **belief system** as a tower of blocks. The bottom block is the key, or bottom, belief holding the rest of the beliefs; the root of all the other programs above it. Always ask the Creator, 'Which key belief is holding this belief system intact?' You can save hours of time by seeking and clearing key beliefs.

As soon as you have the key belief or program, ask for, or find, the proper replacement programs to install in the void of the removed or pulled programs. Then ask yourself or the client what you have learned from having the program replaced and why it was there in the first place. Understanding why we have a program that isn't in our highest and best interests will help avoid recreating the same energy again.

It is always best to find the key belief being pulled and replaced before the end of the session. In addition, be sure to include feeling work in your belief-work session because the insertion of feelings in many instances will expedite the process of finding the deepest program.

Determining the key belief

When doing belief work on yourself or with a client, ask, 'If there is anything that you could change, what would it be?' Then continue asking questions pertaining to the issue until you have reached the specific or deepest issue. When working with clients, you will know when you are close to the key belief if the person becomes verbally defensive, wriggles, or cries in a subconscious attempt to hold on to the program. Pull, cancel, resolve, and replace the issues as necessary on whatever belief levels you have found them.

The key questions to ask are:

- Who?

- What?

- Where?

- Why?

- How?

When you are working with clients, avoid putting your own programs or feelings into the investigation process. For this reason, always remain firmly connected to the perspective of the Creator of the Seventh Plane when you are in another person's 'space' with your intuitive abilities. If you do this, you will get a clear 'read' on the person. In some instances, the client will loop, hide, or take you in circles with the question/answer scenario. Be patient and persistent to find the deepest program. It may be necessary to ask the Creator, 'What is the deeper program?'

If the client begins to experience discomfort during belief work, continue releasing beliefs until it is gone. With the person's permission, download the feeling of what it *feels like* to be safe from the Creator's perspective. Continue with the session until the person is comfortable and has a peaceful demeanor. In most instances, the digging technique must precede the insertions of feelings or the release of programs. The first thing we should understand is which neuronal connection we need to change.

Why dig for beliefs?

Digging brings us to a realization of what needs to be changed. Once you modify the synapses, you should make sure that you change any associated patterns that might interfere with the new concept, as well. Remember that history- and genetic-level beliefs may also block an insertion of a belief.

Digging doesn't mean asking the Creator what to change and nothing more; it involves self-exploration or discussion, since the simple act of talking about the topic will, in effect, bring the programs into the light of consciousness so they can be released spontaneously. For instance, if you insert the feeling and knowing of how to live joyfully, the body's receptor cells will open the gates of happiness – and, if you're working with a client, they should act differently from that moment on.

—

The key point when digging isn't to focus too much on the idea that the brain is being reprogrammed because the subconscious may attempt to replace the new program with the old one.

—

As you encounter a new program, you'll simply be asking the Creator whether to release it, replace it, or delete some aspect of it. We'll explore the digging methods and processes in more detail in the following chapters, but never replace programs without proper discernment. What might at first appear to be a negative program may actually be beneficial and shouldn't be released randomly.

This process is easy! All you have to do is use the key questions: *Who? What? Where? Why? How?* The mind will then start to dig, accessing information like a computer, and will give an answer to every question. Remember, if you or the client get stuck finding an answer, it is only temporary. Change the question from why to how, etc., until the answer manifests. If there is no answer, ask, 'If you did know the answer, what would it be?'

With a little practice, you will learn how to access the mind's ability to find the answer. At any time in the belief-work process, be open to divine intervention and the Creator giving you the key belief. Remember there is generally a positive aspect to all key beliefs, so be sure to find out the purpose it has been serving and what has been learned from it. Beliefs such as, 'If I am overweight my feelings are safe,' or 'If I am overweight my deepest feelings will stay hidden' is the mind doing its best to protect us from pain.

FEELING WORK

Perhaps due to trauma in childhood or later in life, some people never experience (or lose the ability to feel) the energy of certain feelings. In order to have feelings such as joy, to love or to be loved, or what it *feels like* to be rich, or any other unfamiliar feeling, we must be shown what these feelings 'feel' like by the Creator. This is also the reason why some manifestations fail to materialize – because in order to manifest what we want, a soul mate, wealth, etc., we first have to *experience* what it feels like to have these things. In other words, we have to believe these possibilities exist in the universe to make it possible for them to manifest in our lives.

As I explained in *ThetaHealing,* to download a feeling to someone else you need to:

1. Request verbal permission for the download.

2. Command or request the Creator of All That Is to instill the feeling from the Seventh Plane of Existence.

In ThetaHealing, you can also be your own practitioner and do your own feeling work by calling on the Creator and allowing the feeling download to flow through every cell of your body and through all four of the belief levels. Once this feeling has been experienced, you will be ready to create life changes.

—

I have watched many lives changed by simply downloading feelings from the Creator.

—

What might take people several lifetimes to learn can be learned in seconds. The Creator of All That Is can teach us these feelings on every level, as well as remove irrational fears.

Downloading feelings

When this feeling knowledge is downloaded, it creates awareness, understanding, and comprehension and these feelings can have a dramatic effect on your intuitive abilities and create physical wellbeing.

FEELING PROCESS

Use the following process to download feelings.

1. Center yourself.

2. Begin by sending your consciousness down into the center of Mother Earth, into the energy of All That Is.

3. Bring the energy up through your feet, into your body and up through all the chakras.

4. Go up through your crown chakra, raise and project your consciousness out past the stars to the universe.

5. Go beyond the universe, through layers of light, through a golden light, past the jelly-like substance, which are the Laws, into a pearly, iridescent white light to the Seventh Plane of Existence.

6. Make the command or request, 'Creator of All That Is, it is commanded or requested to instill the feeling of [*name the feeling*] into the person [*name the person*] through every cell of their body; on all four belief levels and in every area of their life in the highest and best way. Thank you! It is done. It is done. It is done. It is done.'

7. Witness the energy of the 'feeling' flow into the other person's space and visualize the feeling from the Creator being sent as a waterfall through every cell of the person's body, instilling the feeling on all four belief levels (core, genetic, history, and soul).

8. Once finished, rinse yourself off with the Seventh Plane of Existence energy and stay connected to it.

Commands to download feelings

Use the following commands to download feelings from the Creator.

'I understand what it feels like to...'

'I know...'

'I know when…'

'I know how…'

'I know how to live my daily…'

'I know the perspective of the Creator of All That Is…'

'I know it is possible to…'

'I am…'

'I do…'

Examples of other commands

- Teach the *definition of* [*insert feeling to be experienced*] through the 'Creator of All That Is' from the Seventh Plane of Existence. For example: I know the *definition* of *trust* through the Creator of All That Is.

- Teach *what it feels like to* (be) [*insert feeling to be experienced*]. For example: I know *what it feels like to trust.*

- Teach *what it feels like to understand how to* [*insert feeling to be experienced*] or *to be* [*insert feeling to be experienced*]. For example: I know *what it feels like to understand how to trust or to be trustworthy.*

- Teach *when to* [*insert feeling to be experienced*]. For example: I know *when to trust*.

- Teach that it is *possible to* [*insert feeling to be experienced*]. For example: I know that it is *possible to trust*.

- Teach the *perspective* of the Creator of All That Is and *how to* [*insert feeling to be experienced*]. For example: I know the *perspective* of the Creator of All and *how to trust*.

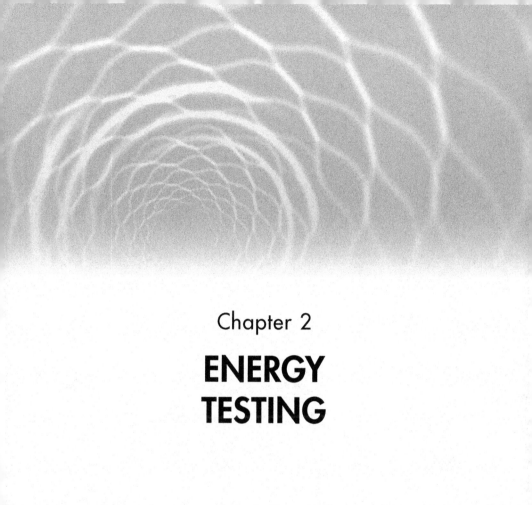

Chapter 2

ENERGY TESTING

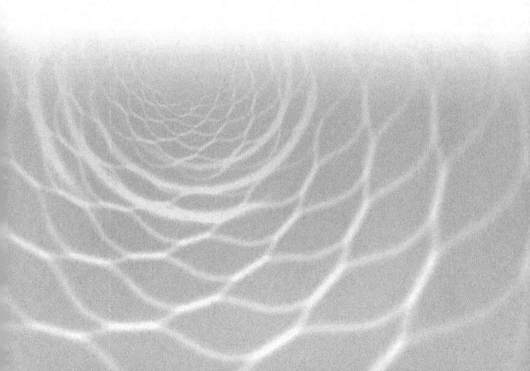

Here follows the correct method for energy testing. I often note that student practitioners don't follow the correct energy-testing procedure, so whether you are a practitioner or working on yourself then I hope you find the following section helpful.

HYDRATION

Before energy testing, be sure that you/the client is hydrated and energetically zipped up. At one time, I thought that I couldn't be energy tested, but after seven glasses of water I could energy test for programs. Energy testing only works if you are fully hydrated and the following key points are worth noting:

- Blood pressure, asthma medication, and caffeine can all affect hydration, so drinking water before a session can make a big difference in the energy-testing procedure. For optimal hydration, add a pinch of salt to your glass of water.

- If having drunk water you are still not hydrated, place your hands on your kidneys (located on the back, below the ribcage) to activate the body into hydration.

- Alternatively, my favorite way to hydrate is to go up to God and ask to be hydrated for energy testing.

ENERGY-TESTING METHODS

There are two methods of energy testing, depending on whether you are working with clients or alone:

Method 1

If you are a practitioner, have the client hold their thumb and finger tightly together and test 'Yes' when their fingers are closed tightly together and 'No' when their fingers naturally release of their own accord.

When energy testing with this method, you need to be observant and make sure the client holds their fingers tightly together and releases their fingers in a subconscious manner in response to the statements they say.

When you pull the client's fingers to test for a 'Yes' or 'No' response, it is important to pull firmly but not so strongly that you hurt the client. Grasp the client's thumb and finger firmly with both of your hands and pull with steady pressure after the client has stated the belief out loud. Make sure the client repeats each belief that you are testing.

Method 2

This energy-testing method is suitable for working alone or with clients.

Stand to face north. When you say 'Yes' your body should lean forward. When you say 'No' your body should lean backward. If you don't lean at all, then you are likely dehydrated (see above).

ENERGY TESTING SHOULDN'T DEFINE THE SESSION

While energy testing is a useful tool – whether you are a practitioner or working alone – it is better to allow the Creator to guide the session. Some practitioners use energy testing as a means of defining the session, but in belief work, I only energy test at the beginning and end of a session – and generally only three or four times. Instead I allow myself to be guided by the Creator.

ENERGY TESTING WHAT WE BELIEVE

Energy testing is only what we believe to be true, which is why you can't, for example, accurately test for vitamin and mineral requirements. If we need a vitamin, we will lean toward that vitamin, because the body will naturally gravitate to substances that it thinks it needs. So, if you crave chocolate cake, it might indicate you need to supplement with selenium and serotonin. If you crave Twinkies or bakery items, you probably need potassium, so you should eat watermelon instead. In the same way, energy testing isn't a definitive method for finding out what a person needs or what is going on.

The truth is that if the body doesn't know what a mineral or vitamin is, then it won't energy test accurately for it. For instance, you might go into a health food store to energy test for supplements, but it isn't likely that you will ever energy test positive for the mineral molybdenum (a heavy metal used to create alloys in steel). However, molybdenum is used in small doses as a supplement to relieve the body of a waste product which causes an overabundance of a yeast called acetaldehyde.

Another way to explain this is with a personal story. Since my body doesn't break down potassium correctly, I will always test that I need it. However, I can't take potassium as a supplement, but need to get it through eating the right foods – such as bananas.

This is why it is easy to energy test positive for 50 different herbal combinations, but herbals work better in simple forms

– using only one or two herbs at a time. (It is also my opinion that herbs shouldn't be used continually, and usage should only be for a few months at a time.)

In addition, the client–practitioner rapport can also affect the accuracy of energy testing. To demonstrate, I used to put turpentine in a cup and have one of my students hold it. Then I would energy test them to see if they needed it and sure enough, because they trusted me, they would give a 'Yes' response.

This is why you should get used to going up and asking God what you need. And, in the case of supplements and other remedies, it is your responsibility to make sure that these have no interactions with any other drugs being taken.

AVOIDING THE ISSUE

When working with clients, ask them to hold their fingers tightly together as you test for the response. However, be careful not to pull their fingers too firmly or too softly, as this can also change their response.

It is also worth being aware that some people will attempt to avoid the issue by influencing the energy testing – particularly if the subject matter is sensitive to them. So observe the client carefully to ensure that they aren't trying to open or close their fingers in an attempt to manipulate the procedure. If this happens, gently make the client aware that they are attempting to change the outcome of the digging session and energy test them again. Tell the client to hold their fingers tightly together as you test for the response.

RAPID EYE MOVEMENT

When working with clients, keep your eyes relaxed and allow them to move naturally as if you were having a dream. It isn't necessary to have rapid eye movement, with your eyes rolling back, in order to get into Theta state or to change someone's beliefs – and can make clients feel uncomfortable.

EYES OPEN, EYES CLOSED

Some clients energy test differently when they have their eyes open because of the different functions of the brain. When the eyes are closed, the person is more relaxed and connected to their subconscious. When the eyes are open, the person is in fight mode. You can still download the client with their eyes open but ask them to close their eyes before energy testing for a belief.

To determine whether you have cleared the key belief or program, energy test the client with their eyes closed. Continue to ask the Creator for the key belief and remove the program, then retest the client with their eyes open and closed.

No matter which energy-testing method you use, you can only energy test correctly with the eyes closed.

ENERGY BUBBLE: CROSSING OVER THE ENERGY FIELD

It is useful to understand that we are very sensitive to our body's 'energy bubble' or 'aura field.' We each have an electromagnetic bubble around us and are sensitive to someone breaking this field. So, when you are working with clients, take care not to allow your body movements to interfere with the client's energy field by 'crossing over' the mid-section of their body in some way – as this can have an effect on the belief-work session.

This is also why it is best to sit offset or directly in front of a client because that way you won't interfere with the aura field when energy testing. You should also 'zip up' the client's aura field with your hand, in a flowing up-and-down motion in front of them, to repair any openings in their space.

PROGRAMS EXPRESSED OUT LOUD

Whether you are working alone or with clients, you can't energy test correctly without saying each and every belief program out loud as a verbal statement. In the same way you can't energy test by simply thinking a belief as it won't give the correct answers. If you/the client doesn't repeat each belief out loud, the energy testing is void for any belief that wasn't verbally expressed.

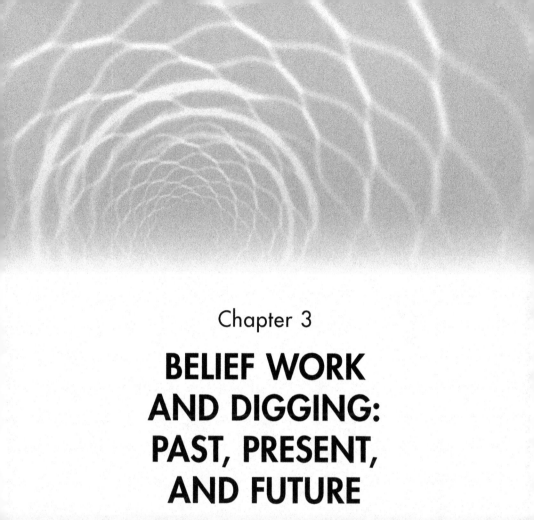

Chapter 3

BELIEF WORK AND DIGGING: PAST, PRESENT, AND FUTURE

When you walk up to your friend and say, 'Let's go to the movies,' this means you are projecting yourself and your friend into the future. When your friend says, 'I need like, a minute and half.' What does this mean? Think about the statement, 'a minute and half'…

This simple, everyday statement means your friend is in the present and projecting into the future at the same time. What this implies is that in everything we do and say, what makes us who we are – our past, present, and future – is all about the illusion of the passage of time. Our brains are hardwired to accept reality this way.

I have people come to my class and say 'Vianna, I am only living in the now, I don't have to remember the past.' But really, everything we do is about our past experiences and previous history. The whole world is based on the history of the past.

We learn from what we have done, what our parents did, what everyone else has done before us, and how these actions continue to affect us in the now and so create the future.

When people say, 'I live in the now, not the past or future. I don't live in the present, I *only* live in the now,' my response is as follows: 'There is no such thing as really living in the now because by the time you realize the "now" it has become the past. The only way you can live in the now is to know what is the past and that you are what is being created in the future. If you want to be a good intuitive and a good healer, you need to be able to create your future. Recreating the future is why some of us are here.'

I think some people read amazing books and take courses which inspire them to focus on where they are in their life. These ideas tell them to enjoy every breath, every second, and celebrate the now. But this doesn't mean losing focus on paying your bills that are coming due in the future or forgetting you are a product of your past actions and experiences.

In the process of belief work, we experience many kinds of belief systems that were created in the past. We find out that much of the reason we do the things we do is because of our past; behaviors which formed subconscious programs when we were children. As we discover these beliefs, we can change certain behaviors and habits as adults for our future self.

The smartest computer that we know of is the human brain. From the first breath you take in the wonderful life-support system that is the human body, your brain starts recording everything that happens to you. Your subconscious runs about 90 percent of your life and, over time, it analyzes things, learns from them, and puts them into a behavior pattern. The subconscious doesn't classify behaviors as 'bad' or 'good,' just as learning experiences.

—

In ThetaHealing, you can't go up and command all your negative behaviors or bad behaviors to be gone. The brain doesn't work that way.

—

For instance, if your mother beat you when were a child while saying, 'I love you,' the brain computes that 'love' can be associated with pain and stress. Therefore, a program may form that it is a little dangerous to fall in love, to have love, or to have someone say, 'I love you.' This is one way that the incredibly intelligent subconscious creates these behaviors.

In ThetaHealing we don't use belief work to take away our past memories but help us to become aware of them, so they can be resolved. Our memories make us who we are and every life experience matters. Digging for beliefs offers us a way to develop an awareness of the past, the present, and the future.

UNDERSTANDING THE PAST

Our genetic-level beliefs form before we are born. Our body's DNA comes from our ancestors and the beliefs they carried – beliefs which helped them in their lives. Decisions made by our ancestors in their present time can then go on to affect their descendants in the future. These beliefs may have been sent down through their DNA and possibly affect the whole being of the descendant.

Our ancestors send down all kinds of genetic information and the best way to sort through it all is with the godsend of belief work. With belief work we can work on the genetic level **seven generations forward and seven generations back**. What is important is to bring forth the good things that our ancestors gave us and magnify them.

Through the centuries, beliefs accumulate in our DNA genetic level. This accumulation of beliefs may affect us now because the past isn't just our past, the present isn't just our present, and the future isn't just our future. We are connected to our ancestors in the past, to our children and relatives in the present, and our descendants in the future in ways that many people don't fully understand.

―

**There is interconnectedness to all things
and this includes our limited understanding
of time as it relates to our DNA.**

―

We learn from our mistakes from the past. But many of the belief systems integrated into our DNA actually serve us. For example, our ancestors learned how to survive, or we wouldn't be here. Among the many skills passed down from our ancestors that we are naturally born with, is the natural desire to help our fellow humans. Helping others is a good survival strategy in a tribal society that had to work together to thrive. This is particularly true if you are a healer of any kind; you have learned that you have an inner desire to help people and probably have this genetic tendency.

Ask yourself: 'What beliefs did you bring down that affect you at a **core**, **genetic**, **history**, and **soul** level?' This question can be answered by doing digging work on the history level.

We believe that we create our own reality. So, in your own reality, ask yourself:

- What are you creating in your life right now? Why are you in your present circumstances?

- Are you in a good situation and are you truly happy?

- Do you get up every day and say, 'I am happy to be alive!'? Do you continue that happiness all through the day, or do you have moments of absolute criticism of yourself and of those around you?

- Do you find yourself going up and down emotionally all day – or at least three times a day? If so, do your emotional ups and downs form a pattern or is every day completely different?

- Are you angry with yourself or with others?

- Are you upset your family isn't what you want?

- Are you upset that a friend or someone else hurt you?

How you answer the above questions may have something to do with your genetic programs and is hardwired from generations of our ancestors having the same patterns. Many people come from families that instill the same beliefs systems that have been taught for generations. Changing these ancient patterns comes when your soul essence recognizes the need to change your beliefs.

BECOMING AWARE OF PROGRAMS FROM THE PAST

When I talk to my ThetaHealers who have worked on their beliefs for a very long time, they are often absolutely convinced they have cleared up every negative belief – which is true because our brain doesn't think everything is negative. They think they have done all the necessary belief work and so don't understand why life still isn't going the way they want. They tell me, 'I have done all my belief work. I don't know what I am doing wrong.' What they are forgetting, however, is they have worked on their present and future, but not their past. Their past isn't only about them, but is also affected by their ancestors' beliefs.

You may have a belief that you are afraid to trust anyone or that life is filled with sadness or you are always ready to fight. Why do you have these beliefs? What is carrying them inside you or why do you have a tendency toward them?

Belief work example one

Client: 'I always have to fight for everything.'

Vianna: *'When did this begin? When did you first have this feeling that you always have to fight?'*

(This client was like many others when I asked this question; he went back into the past for a minute before speaking.)

Client: 'Oh, I don't remember, it's always been there.'

Vianna: *'Well, if you did remember, when did it start?'*

Client: 'It started when I was two, I remember my brother coming in and beating me up, and if I let him beat me up without fighting back I would get in big trouble – physically, mentally, and emotionally – so I learned how to fight.'

Vianna: *'Is this really when it started?'*

Client: 'Yes, I think so.'

Vianna: *'What did you learn from this and what did you achieve from it?'*

(This is all coming from the past when the client was a child, although sometimes people will go deeper than childhood experiences.)

Client: 'I learned that I had to fight for what I believe in.'

Vianna: *'Where did you learn that?'*

Client: 'I don't know, I just remember always fighting.'

Vianna: *'Well, what kind of memories do you have about it?'*

Client: 'My grandfather fought in the Civil War on the Union side. My grandmother was on the confederate side, so there was never peace between them.'

If you start asking these types of questions over and over again, people will walk themselves into the past to their ancestors' beliefs. We may also come up with answers that are much deeper than this time and place, and so it can help to understand our own genetics. If you don't know your DNA admixture then you can get a DNA test to find out how it relates to your ratios of European, Asian, African, and Native American heritage. Once you have this information, you can use it to help unlock your ancestral beliefs.

Other ways that can help us go deeper into the history level is with a **crystal layout**, which can help to uncover where these different patterns started. You don't have to remember where or how the pattern started to realize that it came from your ancestors. Then you can ask: 'Does this belief serve me now?' You may discover it doesn't.

ANCESTRAL PREJUDICE

One thing that doesn't serve us on this Earth is prejudice, but we can carry ancestral prejudices that go back hundreds, even thousands, of years, and are no longer helpful to us in modern life. Yet these prejudices are often buried so deep inside the unconscious they are on a genetic level. As you start digging you see how the past, present, and future are all interconnected. And all that it is necessary to learn is compassion, kindness, and the ability to communicate; these are the things that will help the planet in the present and future.

To identify ancestral prejudice, you might start by asking, 'What would happen if you weren't prejudiced?'

The client is likely to respond along the lines of, 'These people could take me over.'

In response, you might say, 'Is this your feeling or is it coming from something else?' Then energy test for the following programs:

'I am prejudiced against this race.'

'I am afraid that I will be taken over by this race.'

'I am afraid this race will destroy me.'

If the energy test is positive for these or similar programs, they likely come from the past and can be changed.

THE EYES: A WINDOW TO GENETIC BELIEFS

Many issues with the eyes can also be old **genetic beliefs** that you are carrying unconsciously. The eyes are the windows of the soul and if you start clearing up any related beliefs then your eyesight can improve too.

The following are some beliefs that can be associated with the eyes. Energy test for these programs aloud with your eyes closed:

'I see things only the way I want to see them.'

'People deceive me.'

'I feel hopeless.'

'I feel loveless.'

'No one really knows me.'

'No one can really see me.'

'I am invisible.'

'I am my past mistakes.'

'Revenge consumes me.'

'I am afraid of the future.'

'I am afraid of the now.'

'I respect and see other people's space.'

'Other people respect and see me.'

'I feel violated by those around me.'

If the energy test gives a 'Yes' response for these programs, you might need belief work. Whether you are working on yourself or with a practitioner, ask the following questions to understand how and when the issue started:

•   When did this belief begin?

•   Did it start recently?

- Did it start in your childhood?

- Did it start by your own experiences or is it something that is just a fact?

If it is a fact as it relates to the person, it is probably genetic, and their ancestors probably had to deal with many deceitful people. For example, if someone has the belief of 'people deceive me,' you should ask, 'When did you first believe that people deceived you?'

The answer may be, 'I felt like I was deceived when I was eight years old.'

When the client understands that they were deceived as a child, they know why they don't trust anyone. They understand they keep bringing people to them that deceive them because this is something they have learned. The next step is to teach them what it feels like to be respected.

If the client says, 'People always deceive me, that is always what people do,' then you know it is an old genetic belief. Some of the client's ancestors didn't know what it felt like to be completely respected. It might be true that they are being deceived, but if they believe *everyone* deceives them, then these will be the type of people they attract.

—

The Earth is filled with all kinds of amazing people, but if you believe they will deceive you, they will come to you like a magnet.

—

Then you can ask: 'Is releasing this belief necessary for you to move forward?' And then test for the following beliefs:

'I can see through people before they deceive me.'

'I can avoid people that deceive me.'

If these programs energy test with a 'Yes' response, the client is learning to avoid deceitful people. If they test with a 'No' response, then reteach the client's cells what it feels like to move on from this lesson with the correct download.

As I described in Chapter 1 (*see page 20*), downloads are a way of transmitting feelings through the Creator and can teach the body and mind different ways of thinking and doing things, as well as aid belief work. It is possible to download an enormous number of feelings and feel better about life as a result, but you should always understand *why* you are creating your present reality.

Belief session 1: Past, present, and future

When we first start doing belief work, we can **energy test** for behaviors, ideas, or certain concepts that the client would like to work on.

Your first query should be, 'What would you like to work on?'

The client might respond with, 'I would like to work on why I can't make any money.'

This is when you can get into contact with the computer part of the client's brain by asking questions using *Who? What? Where? Why? And How?* – as the following example illustrates:

> **Vianna:** 'Why can't you make any money?'
>
> **Client:** *'Because money is evil.'*

The program of 'money is evil' is usually created in the past. Every time you contact the subconscious part of the brain you should ask, 'Why?' Why is this? How did it happen? What? When? Where? In this way, you show the client how to go back into their past and see where these behaviors come from.

> **Vianna:** 'Why do you believe money is evil?'
>
> **Client:** *'Money is evil because only college people have money and college is evil.'*

(What he is saying is that people who go to college have money.)

Vianna: 'What does that mean to you?'

Client: *'Well I wasn't smart enough to go to college, people who go to college have an advantage over me and I was stupid, I was dumb.'*

Vianna: 'OK, where did that start?'

(I watched the client as he went back in his mind.)

Client: *'Well, it started when I was little. My mother always told me that I was stupid.'*

Vianna: 'OK, why do you feel you are stupid?'

(He went back in time.)

Client: *'Because I was a mistake, I should have never been born.'*

Vianna: 'Why should you never have been born?'

Client: *'Because I was an unexpected child. I should have never been born.'*

Right there is the key belief of 'I should have never been born,' and it has nothing to do with money. When you find the bottom belief, bring it into the present time.

Vianna: 'How is this serving you now?'

Client: *'Well, as long as I am a mistake, I really don't have to try. I was a mistake, so I don't have any pressure to be more than that.'*

*(This is where the client's **chain of beliefs** came into the present.)*

Vianna: 'If you change this, what will happen? If we change this and you really are worth something, what would happen?'

Client: *'If I am important, if something happens and it changes my life, then I have to be accountable and do something with my life – but I am afraid of failure.'*

(This is where the client went into the future.)

As you can see the belief work is coming from the past to the present and into the future. If we focused only on the 'now,' the client wouldn't be open for change and growth.

Belief session 2: Future work

Manifesting by its very nature is a means of projecting change or creations into the future. As this relates to belief work, you can offer the client an awareness of what a manifestation will mean to them in the future.

Vianna: 'If you had all the money you ever wanted, what would you create?'

The client thinks about this question and goes into the future with their mind.

Client: *'I would create a huge successful healing center.'*

But as the client begins to create it in their mind, they begin to reflect on what having a healing center really means.

Client: *'If I create a healing center, I would have to stay there all the time. I would have to be there all the time. I would never have my freedom. I would never have time for myself.'*

This is future-belief work using manifesting and the above example shows how the conscious mind helps the subconscious to understand suddenly the consequences of the manifestation and how several outcomes are possible. First, the subconscious may be blocking the manifestation because it perceives it as a threat. Second, the client may have limiting fears and beliefs to work on. Third, they really don't want the manifestation.

—

We put ourselves in certain situations
and circumstances that protect our
wellbeing (on some level).
In actuality, these situations keep us
from moving forward into the future.

—

If you look at the current situation in your life and be in the *present* moment, you can stop to ask, 'How is this situation serving me in the now?' Then you can come up with all the different things that you are learning from it. If you ask, 'What would happen if the situation changed?' then you can *become aware of*, and *work through*, all the fears about what might change in the future.

Fears can begin in the past but are always in the future. The subconscious begins to travel into the future to surmise the most likely outcome. It begins a likely scenario of events it thinks might happen. The mind then goes to work and speculates on the future and thinks: *If this happens, then this will happen and if this happens, this will happen and so on.* By doing this, you face the fear and then pass through it.

PROGRAMS OF CRITICISM

As ThetaHealers, we should explore the belief systems of everything we feel and enact in our day-to-day existence. If you notice you get up in the morning and get mad at your children for not being what you want them to be, you may have inherited a genetic tendency for criticism. However, it is worth remembering that criticism is also one of our natural survival mechanisms because it is necessary for good judgment – to help us to stay safe and be cautious when necessary. In fact, the ability to compare others to our own morality, to our own ideals, and to be able to say, 'This isn't what I want to be' is just one of many amazing beliefs we have learned from our ancestors. But over time being overly critical of ourselves and others can develop into more than just the ability to judge what we don't want to be and become one of the most negative degrading feelings; it is capable of bringing our energy down more than anything else and only serves to keep us in limbo.

So proper judgment is helpful in certain parts of our lives – especially if your job is a movie critic, so maybe you'd want to keep that kind of judgment – but if you are busy criticizing your parents, your family, your siblings, your friends, and so on, you are using enormous amounts of energy that could be applied to healing, creating your world, and your reality. If you ask your brain why you need it, your brain might give you the message of 'If I don't change, I don't have to fail, I don't have to try, I don't have to accomplish anything, I can just stay here in limbo.'

—

One of the foremost beliefs that keeps us frozen in the present is negative criticism of ourselves and others.

—

Some people actually send out a signal allowing other people to criticize them by sending the thought form of 'If I am not doing it right, everyone is going to notice.' Wouldn't it be better to shift this behavior?

Use the following questions to dig for the key belief:

- When did it begin?

- How does it help you?

- What does it do for you, besides keep you in limbo?

- Does it keep you in limbo, so you can rest?

- Does it keep you in limbo, so you don't have to try for a couple of days?

- Does it make you feel good?

As ThetaHealers, we have a way of going in and seeing other people's lives. If you can intuitively see into another person's life, you have learned to live without criticizing them in that moment. When you look inside them, and you don't prejudge or criticize them, you can see their true heart's intention. If we can see the true heart's intention, we would shift completely within ourselves. If we could shift completely, what would happen? (This is the future way of asking a question.)

Well, if we shift completely, we would change so much that we wouldn't want to stay on this planet: we would evolve, we would become a higher life form, and perhaps want to take our family with us. We would become a spiritual essence – a higher spiritual vibration – and leave this world behind. Perhaps you can now see how even tiny behaviors like criticism can anchor us into patterns that anchor us to this Earth, to this existence.

Gossip, spin, and splitting

Gossip, spin, and splitting are all forms of unkind judgment and criticism of others and can prevent us from evolving. I always thought that gossip was taking the truth and distorting it a little bit, but this is actually called 'spin.' Spin is when someone has learned to twist the truth to their benefit and can include splitting people – telling just enough of the truth to make two or more people turn against one another in an attempt to benefit the splitter. Common gossip is anything that might hurt someone else's feelings if they heard it, while malicious gossip is making up mean, unkind lies.

These actions – spin, splitting, and gossip – occupy the mind and indicate a lack accountability and an inability to achieve in life. What is happening in your life? Are you in limbo? Is everything stuck in your life? Are you unable to manifest more money than you absolutely need? How is your mind working for you?

Remember your mind is always working for you. It is always trying to help you. In ThetaHealing, we not only teach *why* you are doing what you are doing, but to have compassion for yourself when you realize your mind isn't being malicious; it is not trying to sabotage you, it is trying to help you.

If gossip and/or criticism is keeping you in limbo, use the following downloads:

'I know how to live without gossiping about others.'

'I know how to live without making malicious gossip about others.'

'I know how to live my life without creating spin about others.'

'I know how to live my life without splitting the people in my life.'

'I know how to have patience for others.'

'I know how to see the truth in others without tearing them apart.'

'I know how to accept others without being like them.'

'I know what it feels like to live without criticizing myself.'

'I know what it feels like to live without criticizing others all the time.'

'I know how to live without being in limbo.'

'I know how to see the truth about others.'

'I know how to stop myself when I start to go into old patterns of criticism.'

PERCEIVING THE FUTURE

If you can't figure out why you have a belief, it's probably ancestral. Then you can ask the question: 'Why did my ancestors believe this?' And you will probably get an answer. Then you can say 'Am I finished with this? Do I need this in my life? What will happen if this isn't in my life?'

At this point you will have completed the different levels in which you can work on a belief. And many ThetaHealers find the bottom or key **history belief** of the past, but never go forward to:

- What would happen if I changed this?

- How is this helping me?'

- If I change this, what will happen?

If you ask these questions, you will have a better understanding of what will happen in the future.

SHIFTING BELIEFS

We don't always have to do belief work to change a belief because often, when we recognize we have a habit, our brain can change it. The brain works like a perceptive computer and will change habits when it sees that it is necessary – and does this all the time. For example, someone who repeatedly has abusive relationships may recognize they keep repeating the same pattern, and then find a partner that really loves them because the lesson about abuse has been learned.

But in belief work, we can shift beliefs much faster by going up into a Theta brainwave, locating the belief, and changing it quickly and efficiently. Shifting a belief means we discover the pattern is no longer necessary in some way, but don't necessarily release and replace it – because it might be a learning experience from the past that has some kernel of value to it. One of the biggest mistakes people make in ThetaHealing is simply releasing beliefs, before understanding how it has helped and served them.

A good example of this is the belief of, 'I took an **oath** of poverty.' Many people become inspired to command all oaths of poverty to be gone. But changing all past oaths in this way will attempt shift everything, forward and backward in history. This means that if someone in our past history is also learning this lesson, the belief will come back. If you energy test positive for the program of 'I have an oath of poverty' then the answer is to go up and command, 'This oath has been completed' and then you can move forward. This shifts the belief rather than releasing it.

Shifting beliefs is about finally being able to understand your past, present, and future; understanding where the beliefs come from and how they help you to understand yourself. Nothing in life is without meaning.

—

**Everything has meaning. Everything
you have done, everything you have
experienced, makes you who you are.**

—

Use the following downloads to help you move forward:

'I know what it feels like to live without being stuck in the past.'

'I know what it feels like to embrace my past, present, and future to move forward.'

'I know how to understand my past, present, and future to create a better reality.'

'I know what it feels like to be important to my ancestors.'

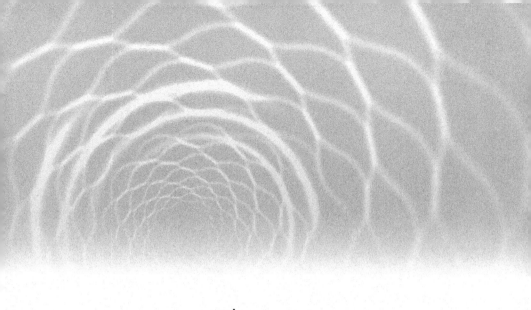

Chapter 4

THE PRINCIPLES OF DIGGING

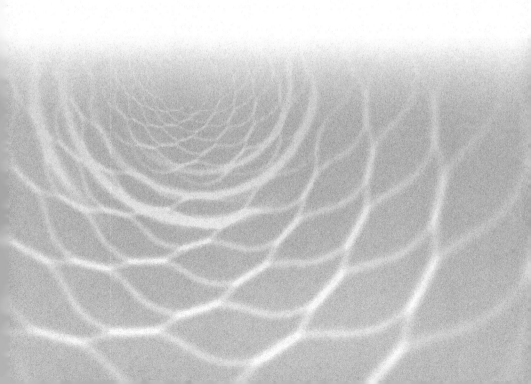

In this chapter we'll be covering the principles of digging for the key or bottom belief.

1. DOWNLOADING BELIEFS

There are some shortcuts to digging for the key or bottom belief, but many practitioners avoid digging work and instead use only downloads in a belief-work session. Downloading feelings is a healing art used in belief work to introduce any feelings that are required. But downloads are only *part* of belief work and won't always release the key belief.

As you listen to the client's statements, they may of course indicate the need for downloads. Some good indicators are when a client says, 'I don't know what that is' or 'I don't what that feels like.' Downloading feelings can then help pierce the bubble or shield that the subconscious has made around the key belief, as described in the Introduction – but may not release it. Downloading feelings is helpful but digging for beliefs is more effective to the overall healing process.

As described earlier in the book, downloading beliefs is useful because the subconscious mind doesn't easily let go of beliefs if it thinks they are serving a purpose. While it is sometimes better to download a feeling to help free the belief over time in order to bring it into conscious awareness, so it can be released, you *must* still find the key belief – and its purpose – to be certain it has been changed.

—

Remember every negative belief is attached to a positive belief and so also needs to be changed.

—

2. LANGUAGE

Some core beliefs may have been created in a different language from the one being used today. For this reason, make the command or request to replace a belief or download a feeling in every language ever spoken – both in the client's mother tongue and those ever spoken by their ancestors. There only needs to be one universal command for every language.

Example of the command: 'Creator download this client in every language that they have ever spoken.'

This means that the download is going into the client's space.

3. MULTIPLE-PERSONALITY BELIEF WORK

When working with people with a multiple-personality, or dissociation, disorder, never command that the personalities integrate into one person. To do belief work simply download them on every personality.

4. DON'T, ISN'T, CAN'T, AND NOT

Many psychologists believe the subconscious doesn't understand the words 'don't,' 'isn't,' 'can't,' and 'not.' So, in order to get an accurate response, avoid using these auxiliary verbs in belief-work process and tell the client to omit these words from their statements. For example, a client shouldn't use a statement such as 'I don't love myself,' or I can't love myself.'

To test properly for a program, the client's statement should be 'I love myself, no' or 'I love myself.' Then you can energy test negatively or positively for this program with a 'Yes' or 'No' response. If the client needs the program to be changed, you can replace 'I love myself, no' with 'I love myself.'

Although many psychologists believe that the subconscious doesn't understand these words, I think that many people *do* understand the difference subconsciously. However, there are many people who do not, so it makes sense to avoid using these words when first starting to do belief work.

5. START THE DIGGING WORK BY ASKING KEYWORD QUESTIONS

Start the digging work by asking questions using the following keywords:

- Who?

- What?

- Where

- How?

- When?

These are the keywords for questions that the client uses in a digging session. 'When did this start?' 'How did this help you?' 'Who was with you?' This will help you not only to look for the negative beliefs but also show how they are serving the client.

6. ULTIMATE TRUTHS: BELIEFS THAT CAN'T BE CHANGED

There are some beliefs that cannot be changed that are called **ultimate truths**. Here are some examples:

- The practitioner cannot program someone to believe that the sun won't come up tomorrow or that the Earth will stop turning.

- The practitioner cannot program someone to be a dog.

- The practitioner cannot change another person's free agency or **free will**.

- The practitioner cannot program another person to love someone when they don't.

For example, one of my students had a belief that she was Joan of Arc and I noticed it caused challenges when the student was paired up with another student during belief-work practice.

I asked them, 'What's going on?'

The student in the role of practitioner told me, 'We are working on why she has to suffer all the time. She believes that she is Joan of Arc. No matter what I do, I can't change this belief.'

The practitioner couldn't change this belief because it was a truth in some way. It may be that the student was genetically related to Joan of Arc or had some kind of connection with her. Instead of pulling the belief of 'I am Joan of Arc,' the practitioner needed to change the associated programs around the energy of 'Joan of Arc' that wasn't serving her, such as 'I have to die to serve God' or other similar programs.

If she had to suffer due to believing 'I am Joan of Arc,' then the negative aspects could be shifted without wasting time working on something that she believed to be true. This belief only needed to be downloaded and then she could get on with her life.

In the same way, if someone energy tests positively that their spouse is cheating on them, it could be due to a lack of trust and needing to work on their beliefs. Cheating might mean that they are dishonest in some way, but it doesn't necessarily mean they are having an affair with another person. The psyche is telling them that something is wrong, but the truth is something that needs to be verified. It could also be that their intuition is right and their spouse is cheating on them.

If after working on the beliefs the client still energy tests positive for the same issue – and their spouse is actually cheating – then the energy test will always give a positive response.

Finally, it's important to note that you shouldn't attempt to pull and replace an ultimate truth such as, 'What doesn't kill you makes you stronger,' because this is actually a *beneficial* belief system of the immune system and it will always replace itself.

One person's truth

One of my more challenging students came to me and said, 'I have the belief that "I have to prove myself to you." I change it, but it comes back.' He was always attempting to push his will on others and I admit I was afraid to let him teach, and when I energy tested myself, sure enough, I had the belief that he had to prove himself to me. This was my truth projected on him, which he was accepting. So, I changed my belief to 'He has to prove himself to God.' I also changed this belief in myself as it related to all my students, knowing that my job was only to teach them.

7. NOT ALL BELIEFS NEED TO BE CHANGED

Not all beliefs need to be changed. I have students come to me and say, 'Vianna I want to pull my stubbornness.' In such cases, I always suggest not to change this attribute because it could also be one of their best traits. Why? Because stubbornness makes a person who they are; they had to be stubborn to get where they are now.

By the same token, you can't pull getting angry or being fearful. Anger has a positive aspect when the brain sends alarm signals in times of danger. Everyone gets angry or fearful from time to time because these are both human survival reflexes. However, it is possible to release an obsession with anger or specific fear phobias that don't serve us.

By way of another example, I had a friend who was an obsessive compulsive and wanted to be healed. However, this precise quality made her awesome at doing paperwork, so I suggested that she needed to keep part of the belief and alter it to serve her.

As a Capricorn, one of my best traits is that I am bossy: I expect things done yesterday and I'll do it myself if I have to; this also makes me a really good boss. I can see what needs to be done and I can multitask. I married a bossy Aries man who, like me, thinks he is always right, and we make a great team. I also have a wicked temper that I keep under good control, but my husband Guy can still find it – it's amazing and I think he likes it. I don't want to change having a temper, I just want to control it and reserve it for emergencies, so I see it as a quality that I don't want to change. I want to be nice and kind but also know when not to be.

—

**What you think is your worst quality
can be altered slightly to be your best
without changing a single belief.**

—

8. VERBAL PERMISSION FOR DOWNLOADS

Sometimes practitioners say that other people have attempted to download feelings without their permission. But this goes against the law of free will; the students are merely being psychic and feeling the negative thoughts of others. Remember negative thoughts can't affect us unless we give the other person our permission or accept the thought-form. I also believe that karma exists in some instances and treating others badly can come back to you, but others can't download or curse you without your permission.

For example, I had a teacher working in another country who said she would curse her students if they went to another teacher. Of course, she did this to instill fear into her students and protect her practice. Once her students realized that she couldn't curse them, they left her – but a small amount of fear remained. Have I corrected her? Of course I have. Has she stopped doing this? Yes. But the damage has been done. The old students tell the new students what she did and the energy of it goes on and on. It is a pity, because this woman is a pretty good healer. Now, there may be some people who can curse others, but it can never harm you when you send it to the light.

> ## ~ IMPORTANT REMINDER ~
>
> Always remember that the person receiving belief work must give you their full verbal permission to remove and replace programs. We have the free agency to keep any belief programs we choose. Another person can't change those programs without our verbal permission. It won't work.

9. DOWNLOADING TO OBJECTS

As well as downloading feelings and beliefs to your subconscious, you can also download enriching qualities into objects in your home and office so that they surround you with positive vibrations. Any inanimate object can be downloaded with a positive attribute to enhance your life, but you will only be affected by the object if you have the receptor for the given program or feeling. For example, if I download my couch with the attribute of being comfortable, the person that sits down on it needs to know what comfort is in order to experience the couch.

While there are also some inanimate objects that won't take a download, such as jade, you always need to ask the object if you can download to it first – because everything in existence has free will. There are times when some objects will refuse the download, but 99 percent will because they accumulate energy by their very natures.

—

**You can't download to food or objects
to effect people in a negative way, as the
object or person will reject it. Any object
can only be downloaded to enhance
the qualities that it already has, not
negative programs that it doesn't.**

—

10. BAND-AID BELIEF WORK

Many practitioners use what I call 'band-aid beliefs' in a session or on themselves. This is when they use downloads instead of digging for key beliefs, as illustrated in the following example.

I might be driving down the road and think, 'I'm so stupid, I forgot to do that.' I realize I am calling myself stupid and know this is something I need to change – something that might be blocking me from being the person I need to become. This might take some belief work to find out where it began, but I don't have time at that moment, so I download 'I am smart, intelligent, and I am doing great.'

These downloads don't take long and can assist me in some way. But the truth is I need to find out *where* the negative program started and *how* it is or isn't serving me, and how it served me before, in order for it to clear completely. So, any time that you don't complete the belief work, this is called 'band-aid' belief work. Once you have time, allocate some space in your life to dig deeper and clear any self-limiting beliefs.

11. NEGATIVE PROGRAMS

The subconscious doesn't know the difference between a negative and positive program or download, so we can't just command that all negative programs be gone instantly. Always remember that it is the conscious mind that makes the decision between a negative or positive program or download.

12. DOWNLOADING NEGATIVE PROGRAMS

The subconscious is also smart in that it won't accept negative downloads 99 percent of the time, but never say yes to one. The subconscious doesn't always know the difference between downloads and negative or positive beliefs, therefore it isn't a good idea to download them. If the subconscious mind accepts a downloaded negative feeling, that is exactly what it will create. It is the conscious mind which makes the decision between negative or positive programs or downloads.

Even some programs – which we might at first think are positive – can have a strange effect. For example, downloading the program of 'I know how to live off nothing,' when what you really want is abundance. The same is true of downloading the feeling and knowing of 'I know the perspective of depression from the Creator of All That Is,' as that is exactly what you will get – *the absolute pure essence of depression*. Even if you follow up with, 'I know what it feels like to live without depression,' or 'I know how to avoid depression,' the subconscious may attempt to create the depression regardless. Your subconscious rejects these kinds of weird downloads 99 percent of the time, but it can still be confusing and unnecessary.

To the Creator, we have the free will to experience life as we choose and will get exactly what we ask for. This is why we should avoid downloading negative feelings in an effort to create a positive result and use a positive feeling instead. For instance, a much better-feeling download might be 'I know how to live without being depressed,' or 'I know what it feels like to live without depression.' It is also a good idea to avoid downloading programs that are similar to 'I know what depression is' or 'I know what abuse is.'

There is always a positive reason why the subconscious holds on to a negative key belief. This is because the subconscious can't separate negative or positive beliefs into categories – and why we can't command all beliefs to be pulled at once. A negative belief serves a purpose in some way and is always held in place for a positive reason. Instead, you should ask, 'What do they get out of having this belief?'

For example, a client might say, 'Everything that I do fails.'

To this you should respond by asking: 'What did you learn, achieve or get out of having this belief?'

To this the client might reply: 'As long as I believe that I will fail I don't have to try, I can stay where I am, and I am safe.'

13. POSITIVE DOWNLOADS WITH A NEGATIVE RESULT

There are some downloads that might be considered positive but have weird effects that cause stress. An example of this might be, 'I know how to deal with conflict.' To the universe this means that you must learn how to deal with conflict. This download will likely bring conflict since that is exactly what you are asking to learn.

When I was a little girl I always avoided confrontations because I was afraid of hurting other people's feelings and this is also why I didn't know how to say 'no.' But when I downloaded myself with 'I know how to deal with confrontations,' I found I had more confrontations than ever before. The correct way to download this program would be, 'I know when and how to deal with confrontations easily.' Now I know that, dealing with any confrontation at the beginning of an interaction, and knowing when and how to say 'no,' saves a lot of time.

Another example might be downloading patience. Are you going to bring situations where you need patience in order to learn how?

But if you download already having patience then there won't be as many weird situations to teach you how to have it. In other words, if you download abilities that have to be practiced before you have them, they can be practiced in a more positive way if they are downloaded in the right way and with the right energy. For example, the right way would be 'I know how, when, and it is possible to be patient in the now.' (This will eliminate stress.)

To give another example, I once experienced pure joy and bliss for seven days without any anger, depression, criticism, or irritation – just perfect joy. Nothing bothered me at all until the seventh day when I wondered if there was something wrong with me and then it stopped; the joy was gone. To find out why the joy was gone I did self-belief work with the Creator and downloaded myself that, 'It is OK to be joyful, constantly.'

As you achieve virtues, you will find that your abilities grow likewise. Your soul is actually inspired to learn kindness, joy, and patience. But when you download these feelings, use the energy of the words, 'I already know how to have patience, kindness' and so on. After downloading these virtues, it is still necessary to practice them to teach the mind how to use them automatically.

14. IMPOSING BELIEFS

Not everyone that visits a healer is going to want to do digging work, but they will likely need it. While doing a reading, you will see whether the client has belief issues, but it is also important to avoid imposing your beliefs on them. Using the correct procedure for energy testing and ensuring the client repeats the statement aloud will prevent this from happening (*see page 33*). This is because we only energy test correctly when we say the statement of the program aloud. Thinking the thought and then energy testing without expressing the belief verbally doesn't work, as the following example illustrates:

One of my students was very upset because she 'supposedly' found out that her father had molested her as a child.

Vianna: 'How did you find out that this happened?'

Student: *'I energy tested for it.'*

Vianna: 'You actually spoke the words aloud of, "My father molested me as a child?"'

Student: *'No, the practitioner "thought" the program to me and said I energy tested positive for it.'*

Vianna: 'Let me energy test for this program. Say, "My father molested me" aloud and close your eyes when you say it.'

She tested with a 'No' response for the program, so I took her into a crystal layout (into a trance state to her childhood). She didn't have any issues from her past and could continue loving her father as she always had.

15. WHEN A CLIENT SAYS, 'I DON'T KNOW'

When someone says 'I don't know' in a session, the statement can mean several things. Some clients will go in circles saying, 'I don't know' to every query. This can mean:

- They are truly at a loss as to how they feel.

- They are avoiding a sensitive subject or their subconscious is protecting the key belief.

- They truly don't know where a belief has come from.

If someone says, 'I don't know' during the digging process, ask, *'But if you did know?'* This question will stimulate a response from the client that may lead to the key belief.

If this doesn't work, this is your cue to attempt to download feelings the client may not know such as, 'I know what it feels like to be safe' or 'I know what it feels like to be loved.' This may help to guide you to the key belief.

16. WHEN A CLIENT DOESN'T HEAL?

We work with medical practitioners to bring about healing but sometimes people hold on to a disease or a belief because they believe healing is impossible or for another reason. For example, I once had a student who did three successful healings after they learned ThetaHealing. The first three sessions worked and the last one didn't, and because of this the client said, 'I am done with ThetaHealing, it didn't work.' However, the following reasons can also prevent a client from healing:

- The practitioner not being kind or showing concern.

- The practitioner being afraid of the disease.

- The practitioner's ego.

- The practitioner projecting their own beliefs rather than the other person's.

- The practitioner feeling hurt when the other person doesn't immediately heal.

- The practitioner being attached to the outcome of the session.

—

**To me it is worth it if one in 10 people heal.
If you change someone's beliefs and let
them know that God loves them then
it is a healing. And if someone isn't
healing then clear your mind and ask
God why the healing isn't working.**

—

I know immediately if the healing is going to work when the client says, 'I have (*for example, this disease*) and there isn't anything anyone can do.' Another statement is 'The only way I can get better is to have an operation.' Then I will do a healing for them to have a good operation. I can train someone to go deep into a Theta state and they can be the best healer, but if the client doesn't want to get better then there isn't much anyone can do. But, as a healer, if we are always connected to the Creator, then I believe 90 percent of healings will work when the client is receptive to the process.

I also find that working with clients in the Sivananda Ashram helps because they believe they can get better. In these cases, because they believe in healing, I find that I don't have to do belief work; I just do a healing and they get better. We also have to accept the immutable truth that people do die and, as healers, we can help them to go to the light when they do.

17. UNDERSTANDING THE PROCESS

Being an effective practitioner of belief work means allowing the client to recognize the issues for themselves. Even if you don't find the key belief in the session, it is likely that the client's subconscious mind will recognize there is something that needs to change (as long as it doesn't perceive the change as a threat).

18. AVOID THE DRAMA

Avoid becoming emotionally entangled with the drama of the client. Every emotion that surfaces concerns the client, not you. No matter what the client does or says, you must remain neutral in order to help them. This clarity can be achieved by working on our own issues, although I realize this can be difficult sometimes. When I become emotionally entangled with a client, I go to the Creator and I ask for the feelings of love and compassion because this is different from emotional entanglement.

There will be times when a client comes in for a reading only to become emotional and may even end up yelling at you. This type of experience can quickly put you off balance but, nine times out of 10, it will have nothing to do with you. In these cases, take care to avoid having an emotional meltdown in front of a client, as it will only block you from witnessing the healing. Also, ask the Creator if the client can safely be a close friend before you make them one.

—

Healers have the challenge of staying in a positive, healthy space, often in the most adverse of conditions. In order to take care of others, you first have to take care of yourself.

—

Without even knowing it, you may be treating a client in the same way their negative subconscious is projecting. In thought and deed, in spoken words and in action, we must treat others with intuitive kindness. In order to do this, it is important to know the difference intuitively between your feelings, programs, and beliefs and those of another.

19. CHANGING THE ENERGY

One important thing to remember is that if you don't like your client, then they may not get better. When this happens, the answer is to spend time working on your beliefs as they relate to certain clients.

I once had a client that was unkind to my office staff (who were also my children). So, when I spoke to this particular client, I was resentful of how she had treated my daughter. Frustrated with her lack of progress, I went up and asked, 'God, why doesn't she get better?'

God said, 'You have to like her, Vianna.' So, I worked on my beliefs and the next time she called the office she was pleasant to everyone. No doubt on some level she could sense how I felt and when I changed my beliefs about the situation, hers did too.

20. DUAL BELIEFS

During the digging process, dual beliefs usually clear when you find the key belief. For instance, I had the dual beliefs of 'I am rich' and 'I am poor.' Common sense would say to check for an opposite belief because, after all, my checking account also goes up and down, so I went up to the Creator to ask why.

> **Vianna:** 'Why do I only have enough money to get from one month to the next?'
>
> **Creator:** *'What are you worried about? You always have enough month to month.'*
>
> **Vianna:** 'Why is this?'
>
> **Creator:** *'Money inspires you to do healing. As long as you have to make money you go to work every day. You have to pay your bills, and this inspires you to be a healer.'*

(The Creator didn't tell me it was due to having a dual belief because it is the key or bottom belief that is important.)

> **Vianna:** 'Oh no, Creator, I would still go every day if I had plenty of money!'
>
> **Creator:** *'Really? Last Wednesday you didn't feel well but you went to work and healed a little girl. But if you had plenty of back-up money you would have stayed in bed, so maybe you should learn to be a healer without money being your inspiration.'*

After this belief-work session, I refocused on healing for love and for my financial situation to change. But sometimes belief work doesn't come down to having a dual belief, but 'Why did I create this in my life?' This doesn't mean that people don't have dual beliefs in the digging process, but that you should focus on the underlying or key belief.

One thing that some ThetaHealers say after practicing belief work for a few years is they have done all their belief work and have nothing left to work on. To these people, I say, 'Fine, but without further belief work you won't develop,' because our ego is our worst enemy.

21. RESENTMENT AND GRUDGES

Every person in your life serves you in some way. If one particular person gives you a difficult time and presents resistance in your life, perhaps it is the way they are motivated. Are they motivated by individuals that create resistance in their life? Ask them about the people in their life and how they affect them.

You can also release individual resentments by using belief work but you must also release any related grudges at the same time. You can do this by asking the client if they have a grudge against someone or something that is serving them.

22. GETTING CLOSE TO THE KEY BELIEF

You will know when you are close to reaching the key belief when you (or the client) start to get a little uncomfortable and tired. Your client might say they don't want to continue the belief work or simply give up. This is because it is the subconscious' last chance to hold on to a program which it thinks is helpful. Usually the brain holds on to a belief when that belief is in our history level (*see page 13*).

A good example is doing belief work with someone with breast cancer. At first, the client is all happiness, but as the belief-work sessions continue they may begin to become more difficult and confrontational. When the client starts to act this way, there is a good chance that you are close to the key belief. Anger in a belief-work session can also be an indicator that the client is getting better. When people get sick they often get to the point when they no longer care about getting better and apathy sets in. Anger in this case can stimulate their adrenals, boost their energy, and so make them want to live.

Another indication that you are getting close to the key belief is that the client might begin to get on your nerves. Nevertheless, the key belief should be found before the end of the session or the client may experience a healing crisis. Continue with the session until the client is comfortable and has a peaceful demeanor.

~ **IMPORTANT REMINDER** ~

Don't use a notebook to write notes about your clients. If you are writing down beliefs, you are not being present and working from the heart. This helps clients feel safe and if you become confused or lost during the session, then ask the Creator for guidance.

23. DOWNLOADS INDICATING NEGATIVE BELIEFS

In some instances, as you download a client with feelings, belief systems will be released and even indicate that you have reached a key belief. For example, if you download a feeling, such as 'I understand what it feels like to be gracious and kind,' it might bring up the issue of 'it's dangerous to be too kind' and 'I will be taken advantage of and be hurt.' If this happens the client might reject the download.

In most instances, when you download a feeling, the client will feel euphoric. But if there is an issue which conflicts with the download to the client, the feelings will cause them not to take it. For this reason, as you witness feelings being downloaded, it is best to ask the client how they feel when they accept the new feelings.

In ThetaHealing, we not only isolate the beliefs that need to be replaced, but also add new beliefs. When we isolate the belief and understand how it is serving us in the present then we can look to the future and see if this is something we need, if this is something we can change, and how to change it.

Belief work is always past, present, future; it is always working on why we are what we are and how to understand ourselves.

24. CELLS TALK TO CELLS

We know that cells in the body are interconnected and communicate with one another through an inexplicable language that isn't clearly defined. For this reason, it is also possible for cells to communicate with the cells in another person's body through projected thought. This transmission works in the same way that we are all interconnected through the All That Is energy. In this way, the essence of pure thought can be projected through physical touch to communicate cellular information – such as how to visualize, send consciousness, or create healings – provided the body doesn't perceive the message as a threat (which is often the case, if the client has experienced sexual or physical abuse, because touch has to be consensual).

When communicating on a cellular level, it is important that you are in a Theta state. When you touch the client's hand in a Theta state of mind, I believe the essence of cell knowledge is immediately transferred as a message into their cellular knowledge. This message automatically puts the client into a Theta brainwave with you, and thus in a conducive state to accept healings.

Although it is worth noting that it generally takes at least one **sleep cycle** for all the information from the cells to be understood by the brain. And also, that cellular healing doesn't replace belief work, feeling work, or digging processes because the client must be consciously aware of the feelings and programs that they accept.

25. THE ART OF SELF-BELIEF WORK

Doing belief work and digging for yourself takes a little bit of discipline, but both the following methods are effective in uncovering beliefs.

BELIEF WORK METHOD 1

Using this process means you can easily search for the key belief for yourself by being both practitioner and client. Imagine sitting in front of yourself, talking to yourself while connected and talking to the Creator and energy testing for programs. When working with yourself, just as in a session with a practitioner, you must say each program out loud. You can do this by going directly up to the Creator and asking:

- When did this start? Show me when this started.

- How old was I when this happened?

- Does it go deeper?

- How is this helping me and what did I learn from it?

- Why did I create this?

- How is it helping me?

- What virtue am I learning from it?

- Creator, what do I replace it with?

Ask these questions and receive the answers you need.

In any belief work you always connect with the Creator because it is one of the most valuable things that you can develop as a healer. You always ask the Creator where the belief is taking you. Please understand that you can go up and ask God if you have a belief and you should hear a 'Yes' or 'No' response. For instance, if you ask God why you are sick all the time, you might get the response of: 'Because when you are sick you don't worry about all the things in your world. You don't have to worry about your business, your children as much. You can focus on yourself and you are using this to avoid being stressed.'

BELIEF WORK METHOD 2

In this process, stand to face north. When you say 'Yes' your body should lean forward. When you say 'No,' your body should lean backward, indicating a negative response. If your body doesn't lean at all, you are likely to be dehydrated, so ensure that you hydrate and then try the process again. (See also Chapter 2 for the correct energy-testing methods and processes.)

I find that this method is more effective than self-energy testing by holding the thumb and finger tightly together to test 'Yes' or 'No.' This is also a useful method for testing for a program that you don't want to face.

Allow the Creator to guide you

Create quiet time to work with yourself by making an appointment with yourself. We tend to avoid working on ourselves, because the subconscious attempts to take over and tells us, 'Go make dinner' or 'I have to go to work.' This is the way the subconscious avoids the belief work because it believes that it is keeping you safe. And if you tend to 'feel' rather than 'see' things then feeling the answer is just as good as seeing it. I always say that I can train people to see, but feeling is the gift.

One question that I am often asked is how do I tell the difference between the mind and the Creator?

When you go up and connect to the Creator and ask a question, you get an immediate answer. If the answer comes from your mind, you will be told something like, 'It's getting late, I should go cook dinner.' This is not the Creator talking to you; this is you attempting to avoid belief work. The Creator is perfect love and intelligence.

For instance, if you believe that love is pain, you will avoid love. If you attempt to work on it, there might be an internal struggle with the self-belief process. Then you will have to ask the Creator to show you where the belief started. Then you can download what real love is – that it is safe – or change the belief that you have to let people that you love hurt you.

—

**Being consciously aware of your
beliefs is very important.**

—

Doing belief work with myself (which I call self-belief work) takes self-discipline, even for me, but I like going up to the Creator for answers. Working directly with the Creator can also be an advantage over working with a practitioner, who may confuse the issues with what *they* think are your beliefs. In this scenario, you are likely to feel intruded upon and be unwilling to cooperate – and this is also why it is so important for a practitioner to be connected to the Creator in the session. On the flipside, working with an experienced, kind practitioner, who you also feel safe with, can prevent you from trying to hide any deep issues from yourself.

Use the following downloads for self-healing:

'I know that the history of the planet, the history level, the genetic level all matter, and I know how to work on them.'

'I understand what it feels like to know why I do what I do.'

'I know how to understand myself and work on myself.'

'I know how to connect to the Creator and ask, why I have a belief, when it started, how to shift it, what I need to do to change it, what downloads I need, and what I need to shift beliefs in the highest and best way.'

26. OVERCORRECTION

When digging for your bottom or key beliefs, you may experience what is called 'overcorrection.' As you begin releasing deep programs and instilling new feelings, it may bring up family issues. This releasing-and-instilling process is likely to give you a great deal of empowerment and you may have the desire to get on the phone and start screaming at these people. Please give yourself time to process all the feelings that have arisen during the belief-work session before taking any action. Many of these programs will have been created a long time ago and the person who caused them to form within you has likely changed since then. They are not the same person anymore and won't understand why you are screaming at them, and you won't receive any absolution from doing so.

—

**Do your best to refrain from overcorrecting
any situation or issue that you have with
another person until you are balanced.**

—

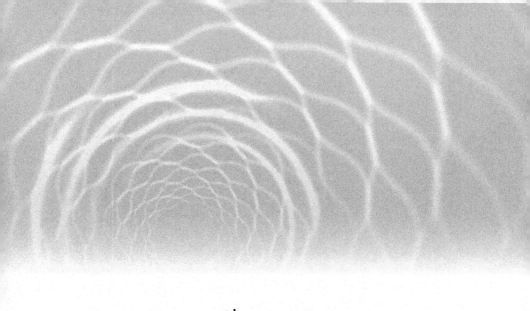

Chapter 5

THE FIVE BASIC STEPS OF DIGGING IN BELIEF WORK

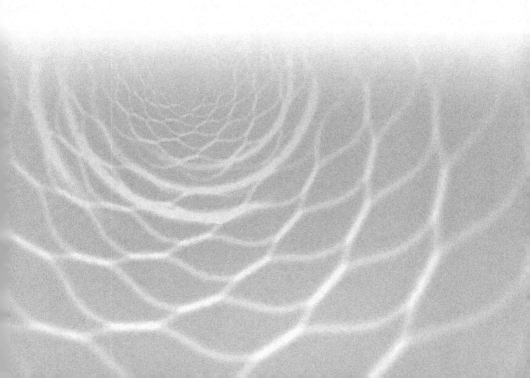

As a practitioner working with clients, there are five essential steps for digging for beliefs, which we'll cover in this chapter before moving on to the more advanced processes in the next chapter:

1. **Establish rapport:** A bond of trust between the client and the practitioner will encourage open communication.

2. **Identify the issue:** This is the issue that the client says they want to work on.

3. **Use basic keywords and questions:** Begin the digging process for the client's key or bottom belief in order to release all the other beliefs stacked above it.

4. **Change the beliefs:** Connect to the Creator and witness the beliefs being changed on all the four belief levels: core, genetic, history, and soul.

5. **Confirm the change:** Confirm the beliefs have been changed by energy testing each belief that has been released and replaced.

Let's go through each of the five steps in more detail:

STEP 1: ESTABLISH RAPPORT

Start by greeting the client and making them feel comfortable. Establishing this bond of trust will encourage open communication between you.

Listen, acknowledge, and question

Listen to what the client has to say and acknowledge it, and then continue to asks questions without being aggressive.

Be open to listening to what the client is saying and be aware of the energy that underlies each statement, because each statement is an indicator of the bottom or key belief. Don't put words into the client's mouth but make them feel what they are saying has validity and value – because it does. Also, each person is different from everyone else in the world so, while there may be similarities in beliefs, each person should be treated as a unique individual.

Make eye contact and read their body language

It is important to make eye contact with the client and watch their **body language** because their physical responses will indicate when a sensitive point in the belief-work dialogue has been reached.

STEP 2: IDENTIFY THE ISSUE

At the start of the belief-work session, ask the client what they want to achieve. There are so many avenues of beliefs to work on but remember the session is about the client: their needs and what they want to work on.

Ask the client, 'What would you like to work on today?'

If the client answers with, for example, 'I would like to work on my issues with my family,' this issue is the client's 'surface belief' and the starting point which may lead to the key belief – the cause of the issue. This belief will likely represent a situation in the client's life that they would like to change.

Energy test

Perform an energy test to determine what the client believes to be true as it pertains to the issue (see Chapter 2 for the correct energy-testing methods and processes).

Be observant and make sure that the client always holds their fingers together firmly and releases them in a subconscious manner in response to their spoken statements. Be careful the client doesn't try to open or close their fingers in a conscious attempt to manipulate the procedure.

Set goals with the surface belief

Set a common goal for the client by saying, for example: 'Let's investigate the issue and get to the bottom of it.' Remember don't take notes in a notepad, as this may cause the client to feel there is something is wrong with them or as though they are being studied or analyzed.

STEP 3: USE BASIC KEYWORDS AND QUESTIONS

In order to use the digging process to find the client's key beliefs, your approach should be one of intuitive exploration Ask the client questions using the following basic keywords to identify their issues and negative beliefs:

- When?

- What?

- Who?

- Where?

- Why?

- How?

Use these keywords to dig for the belief, as shown in the table below:

Keywords	Example
When?	*When* did it happen first?
What?	*What* did you learn from it?'
Who?	*Who* told you this?
Where?	*Where* did this first begin? *Where* were you when this happened?
Why?	*Why* do you think you are sick?
How?	*How* does this make you feel? *How* does it serve you?

Using these keywords correlated with the questions creates an opening to the client's deeper belief programs. From here, there are then 10 different digging approaches, or shortcuts, to identify the key belief – depending on the type of issue being presented. We will cover the 10 digging approaches in more detail in the next chapter.

STEP 4: CHANGE THE BELIEFS

Some of the indicators that you have reached the key belief are that the client will loop, hide, or go in circles with a question-answer scenario. Be patient and persistent to find the deepest belief. In addition, the client may attempt to distract you by changing the subject, and/or become nervous and emotional.

The client may also become emotional, make nervous movements, squirm in their chair, scratch their head, fold their arms, start to get tearful, and their breathing may become erratic. The client may also look down at their feet and not make eye contact. This body language indicates an attempt on the part of the subconscious to hold on to the key belief.

—

If the client begins to experience discomfort while doing belief work, ask them if they would like to download what it feels like to be safe.

—

Changing beliefs through the Creator

I often say I have the easiest job in the world. All I have to do is listen to the Creator and do what I'm told to do. In the same way, your digging process (whether with yourself, another person, or a client) should be practiced from a standpoint of co-creating with the Creator. All you have to do is listen to the Creator.

Throughout the process, be sure to interact with the client from a Seventh-Plane perspective through the Creator of All That Is. This means that the digging interaction comes from the Seventh Plane of Existence, not the Third Plane. Co-creation permits you to get out of your own paradigm and into that of the client. Don't permit your own judgment to influence your investigation in the belief-work session. Remember: the digging process is about the client.

—

A belief-work session is an interaction between the client, the practitioner and the Creator. The Creator is always with you.

—

Ask the Creator

When working with a client, avoid projecting your beliefs or feelings into the investigation process. The best way to do this is to stay firmly connected to the perspective of the Creator. As described earlier, the client may loop, hide or take you in circles with the question-answer scenario. Be patient and persistent to find the deepest belief.

Always ask for the Creator's help when you need extra guidance. Ask the Creator to guide you in your digging session. For example, ask the Creator to tell you the bottom or key belief, what beliefs to energy test, and what feelings to download.

For example, you might ask, 'Creator of All That Is, it is requested that you tell me the feeling to download for this person. Thank you! It is done, it is done, it is done.'

You can also call on the Creator during a belief-work session:

- If you feel unsure, ask the Creator what questions you should ask the client.

- When a client presents multiple issues, ask the Creator which specific issue to focus on first.

- To ask whether a specific belief is a key belief.

- To ask the Creator for the key belief.

- To ask for a new positive belief to replace a negative belief.

- To ask what positive feelings to download into the person that will help in a situation.

You might also ask, 'Creator of All That Is, what feelings does this person need? Thank you! It is done, it is done, it is done.'

You can also *change the* belief and download feelings through *the Creator* by:

- Conducting a healing on any negative beliefs that are found during the session by downloading feelings as needed.

- Making the client aware of the key belief.

- Going up and connecting to the Creator and witnessing the beliefs being changed on all the core, genetic, history, and **soul belief** levels.

STEP 5: CONFIRM THE CHANGE

Confirm that the belief has been released and replaced by energy testing the belief that has been changed (see Chapter 2 for the correct energy-testing methods and processes); this gives both you and the client validation.

As described in the previous chapter, you will know when you are close to the key belief if the client becomes verbally defensive, squirms, or begins to cry. This type of resistance is an attempt on the part of the subconscious to hold on to the key belief. If the client begins to experience discomfort while doing belief work, ask them to download the feeling of what it *feels like* to be safe.

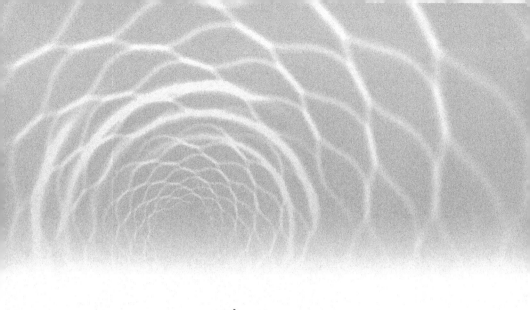

Chapter 6

THE 10 DIGGING APPROACHES (OR SHORTCUTS)

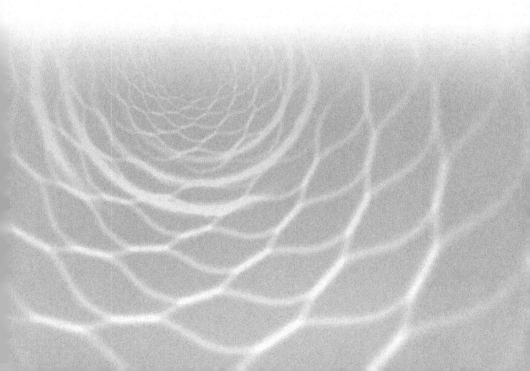

There are 10 digging approaches or shortcuts which you can use to identify the key belief – depending on the type of issue – and all these approaches can be used interchangeably in a single belief-work session.

Digging approach	Description
1. Fear	Identify the deepest fear underlying all the other fears.
2. Resentment	Understand the situation by asking, 'When was the resentment created?' And also, 'What is the reason behind the resentment?' This approach can be used for resentment and any other negative emotions, except fear.

Digging approach	Description
3. Illness 1	Uncover why the illness was created. Ask, 'How is the illness serving you and what good thing has happened since the illness started?'
4. Illness 2	Imagine the illness gone in the future. Ask, 'What would happen if you were completely well?'
5. Manifesting	The client visualizes what they would like to manifest. Ask questions to identify the issues such as 'What would happen if you got what you want?'
6. Genetics	Identify the issue by asking if a certain belief is the client's mother's belief, father's belief, or an ancestor's belief.
7. History level	Work on the beliefs which have been carried forward from past lives and the group consciousness.
8. The impossible	Teach the brain that what seems to be impossible may actually be possible.
9. Present digging – learning from hardships	Creating awareness that every hardship contains a deeper purpose. Ask, 'What benefit are you getting from the hardships that you are experiencing?'

Digging approach	Description
10. Learning virtues	The soul's purpose in this life is to learn virtues and develop abilities. Ask 'What virtues are you developing from your experiences?'

Among the following 10 approaches, fear and resentment are the basic approaches and the building blocks for all the other digging approaches. But remember the approaches described in this chapter are only suggestions to guide your work with clients because no two people are the same and each digging session is going to be different. The digging process is an intuitive exploration and finding the bottom or key belief is an art form; the 10 approaches are therefore simply suggestions to guide your belief-work sessions.

The digging process is the search for the key belief that created the program to release all the beliefs stacked above it. To become proficient at digging work, you must have an understanding of how asking the right questions can identify the underlying key beliefs; the following 10 approaches endeavor to guide you to do this:

DIGGING APPROACH 1: FEAR

In a general sense, there are two different emotional energies that motivate us: fear and love. Love should be the first motivation, but this isn't always the case. Unconditional love is of the highest vibration in the universe and fear is one of the lowest. In belief work, we don't attempt to remove the emotional response of fear because this is a natural human reaction; it is our inbuilt survival response for times of emergency. For this reason, it is important to be able to discern the difference between dysfunctional 'fear programs' and the occasional normal emergency response of fear.

Living in constant fear is a negative program, as are phobias, and this is when fear also causes a problem. Uncontrolled fear can block just about anything and this includes love, while compulsive fears can evolve into phobias. One way to change a phobia is with belief work and finding the key belief which is holding the phobia in place.

—

Compulsive irrational fear accomplishes nothing. The negative energies of fear, doubt, and disbelief are some of the most prevalent blocks that present themselves in belief work.

—

With any intuitive process, fear shouldn't ever enter into the quotient of healing on your part. So, before starting to work with clients, it is important to clear any of your own fears or prejudices.

Instead of witnessing the Creator do the work, some healers become fearful that the process isn't working and decorate (by which I mean embellish) the client's beliefs in the digging process. Decorating can cause the client to go through unnecessary emotions and what could have been finished in 30 seconds can take the client much longer to process.

Start the digging work

Follow the trail of fear beliefs through to the source of the greatest fear by asking key questions to find out why this feeling came about, how this feeling happened, and when it began. These questions will open the client's subconscious mind to their deeper beliefs.

To identify the deepest fear that underlies all other anxieties, ask:

- What are you afraid of?

- What is your greatest fear?

- What is the worst thing that would happen (if you were in a given situation)?

- How did that feel when it happened?

- What would happen next in the situation?

- When was the first time that you felt this fear? When did it begin?

- What is the worst thing that would happen if you were faced with your greatest fear?

So, when digging for fear, the first question is 'What are you afraid of?'

The client responds with, for example, 'I am afraid of water.'

Then you ask, 'What would happen to you because of your fear of water?'

The client says, 'I'm going to drown.'

If the client is afraid of something specific, it is rarely what they are actually afraid of and there is usually an underlying cause to the fear.

If someone is afraid of water the belief will be, 'I am afraid of water,' and you remove this program and replace it with, 'I am not afraid of water,' nothing will change because water isn't necessarily what the client fears; the fear is coming from something else.

At this point you know that water isn't the client's fear but that is how it is presenting. The next step is to follow the fear to the key belief, so the client realizes what they are afraid of.

Practitioner: 'What happens if you drown?'

Client: *'Well, if I drown I will die.'*

Practitioner: 'Then what will happen?'

Client: *'If I die, I will leave my children and if I leave my children then I will be a failure and if I'm a failure I fail God and if I fail God it is wrong for me to go to the light. I will be stuck in darkness.'*

With these statements, the client has done their own digging work. The practitioner used the query keywords of who, what, when, where, how and just listened to what they said.

—

Connect to the Creator and ask questions pertaining to who, what, when, where, and how.

—

Practitioner: 'What will happen if you are stuck in the darkness?'

Client: *'I will be stuck in darkness and I will be in the nothing.'*

The practitioner now realizes that the person isn't afraid of water but of 'the nothing.' As in this short example, when a client gives this much detail it indicates they are remembering an occurrence that is real to them. It doesn't matter where the memory comes from, walk them through it so they are not left in the middle of their greatest fear. In the above scenario, the client's real fear is the 'nothing' and that they have disappointed God and left their children. Which fear is the real one is dependent on how many times the client repeats it.

To change these beliefs, ask the Creator to pull the fear of nothing and replace it with the belief that the Creator tells the client – which is often 'you can always watch your children' and 'you are always loved by the Creator in the energy of creation.' Once you pull the fear of nothing, all the other fears fall apart. Once the fear is gone the client is unlikely to have a phobia of water. To test this, ask your client to imagine being in water and ask them how they feel.

One indicator of a key belief is if the client repeats something over and over, such as 'I'm a failure to God,' or 'I'm a failure to my children,' so listen carefully to what the client says.

The key belief of 'I am afraid of the nothing' is one of the greatest fears of humankind. The 'fear of the nothing' is the apprehension of there being nothing after death, that there is no God, and that we will all come to nothing.

If you reach an impasse with the digging process and don't know which direction to follow, patiently watch the client talk about their feelings about their surface beliefs. It may take the client a little time to sort out where the fear is coming from and they may go back to another time and place to find it.

Continue the digging work

For any negative bottom or key belief, there may be a positive reason that the subconscious is holding on to it. Belief work should always have a positive outcome, which is why it is very important to always find what the client is learning from this belief experience.

When you find the client's key belief, ask:

> **Practitioner:** 'What do you get out of having this belief?'
>
> **Client:** *'Everything that I do fails.'*
>
> **Practitioner:** 'What did you learn, achieve, or of get out of having this belief?'

The above example shows how you can help a client understand that, on a soul level, every life experience has a purpose – even a fear belief.

—

Remember that fear programs can be passed on through the genes or the history level. Pull, cancel, resolve and replace these energies as needed.

—

DIGGING APPROACH 2: RESENTMENT

There is always an underlying reason for resentment. As long as we resent someone, we keep them away from us – even if it is a psychological separation. When we resent, we learn something from the situation or person and we will hold on to resentment as long as we are learning from it.

We also use resentment to keep us on this Earth plane. Resentment is a very heavy thought form, just as love is a lite thought form. When we encompass these lite thoughts, we become more enlightened. Many people have graduated from this Earth plane without leaving it through death. Now we are allowed to remember that we are enlightened and can become enlightened on this plane, even though our subconscious may not be ready for this idea. So, to keep us grounded on this Earth plane, resentment comes in. The Creator says, 'If we can clear the resentment from our mind, we can move things without touching them. Resentment blocks our psychic abilities.'

The feeling of resentment will certainly ground you in this existence, but it will also protect you from the very thing that you resent, so the brain isn't going to release it that easily. For instance, let's say a client resents their father, but if you pull this program and replace it with forgiveness it might last for two or three days.

One of my students sat in the bathtub and pulled all her resentments and the next day she was two pant-sizes smaller.

Another student did the same thing with similar results – but when I attempted this, I didn't lose anything. This is because unless we get to the key belief, which is holding the resentment, the challenge will come back (and the weight).

—

One of the most important things with belief work is to understand that the key belief is generally positive in nature.

—

Start the digging work

For instance, if someone has the following program of 'I resent my father because he beat me.'

If you pull and replace this program, the client may feel better for two or three days but the only way to create long-term change is to find out what is *learned* from it, how it created a positive aspect, and why it is serving them.

Ask the client, 'What did you learn that is positive from your father beating you?'

The client is likely going to argue with you about your query, so persist in asking:

- If there was a *positive result* from this experience what would it be?

- What did you learn from being beaten by your father?

The client may say, 'I learned I would never beat my children.'

At this point in the session, you are dealing with both negative and positive beliefs. Teach the client to keep the confidence that was developed from the negative situation, while at the same time giving a download of what it feels like to receive love without being hurt. Then you can energy test the client to ascertain if they still have the resentment.

Digging session: Resentment

The following approach may be used for resentment and all the other negative emotions, other than fear.

Vianna: 'Who do you resent?'

Client: *'I resent my mother.'*

Vianna: 'Why do you resent your mother?'

Client: *'I resent my mother because she beat me all the time. She would lock me inside and didn't let me play outside. I grew up without being able to play outside. When I was a child I wanted to dance, play music, and paint, but my mother wouldn't pay any money for those things.'*

Vianna: 'Did she have money for these things?'

Client: *'Yes.'*

Vianna: 'So, she never let you be you.'

Client: *'Yes. She lives close to me now, but I try not to communicate with her. She wants to heal her relationship with me, but I keep my distance.'*

Vianna: 'Close your eyes. Tell me, what did you learn from her beating you all those years ago – something that is good that you learned.'

Client: *'I learned to do everything my own way.'*

Vianna: 'What did you learn from being locked behind the glass?'

Client: *'I learned to be able to be alone and do things alone.'*

Vianna: 'What did you learn from not being able to follow your artistic nature?'

Client: *'The only thing I learned from this was not to do it to my child and I tried to give her the opportunity to be artistic, but she didn't want it.'*

Vianna: 'Do I have permission to teach you that you can follow your path without someone beating you? Without someone forcing you to follow a different path.'

Client: *'Yes.'*

Vianna: 'Do I have permission to download you so that you can be comfortable being alone yet with other people when you want?'

Client: *'Yes.'*

Vianna: 'And that you can find your independence without being locked away?'

Client: *'Yes.'*

Vianna: 'Would you like to know how to follow your dreams instead of someone blocking you all the time?'

Client: *'Yes.'*

Vianna: 'That you can offer your children music and art without trying to force it on them?'

Client: *'Yes.'*

Vianna: 'Give me your hand and make a circle with your thumb and index fingers. Now I'm going to energy test you for "Yes" and "No." Say "Yes" and say "No." Say, "I resent my mother."'

Client: *'I resent my mother.'*

(She energy tests with a 'No' response.)

Vianna: 'Say, "I can be free from my mother making my life miserable."'

Client: *'I can be free from my mother making my life miserable.'*

(This is resentment work. But I am not finished yet.)

Vianna: 'Would you like to know what a real mother is supposed to feel like? What a real mother's love is? God's definition of a real mother's love?'

Client: *'Yes.'*

Vianna: 'Would you like to know how, when, and that it is possible to be an amazing mother?'

Client: *'Yes.'*

Vianna: 'Say, "I can work on my mother."'

Client: *'I can work on my mother.'*

(She energy tests with a 'Yes' response.)

Vianna: 'Say, "My intuition tells me that my mother would work better with another healer."'

Client: *'My intuition tells me that my mother would work better with another healer.'*

(She energy tests with a 'No' response.)

Vianna: Say, "I can work on my mother without feeling forced to do so."'

Client: *'I can work on my mother without feeling forced to do so.'*

(She energy tests with a 'Yes' response.)

Vianna: 'Would you like to know what it is like to be able to say no in a good way?'

As you can see we had removed some resentment, but if this were a regular session, this client wouldn't have finished the belief work. I would use all the other digging approaches as needed and continue to work on the client's beliefs of being a healer and a mother.

Continue the digging work

Every belief serves us in some way. Unless you find out why the belief is serving the client, their brain will create it again – even after it has been released and replaced with a new belief. Find the reason behind the resentment and change it, so that the client can move forward and permanently remove the resentment by asking:

- What are you learning from this belief?

- How does it serve you?

- Is this belief keeping you safe?

- How does this resentment serve you?

Example

Practitioner: 'How does this resentment serve you? What are you getting out of it? What are you learning from it?'

Client: *'I learned to excel. I learned to be the best I could be at anything I did to meet my mother's expectations.'*

Example

Practitioner: 'How did it serve you? What did you learn from it?'

Client: *'I learned that I would never beat my own children. I learned how to please myself and be independent. I learned it is safer to be alone.'*

Practitioner: 'Do I have permission to download you so that you can be independent without failing? That you can receive love and that you are safe without having to be alone?'

DIGGING APPROACH 3: ILLNESS 1

Sickness can take a long time to work on because it's easy to get addicted to the drama of it. In addition, when we go up and ask, 'God, how many beliefs need to be changed,' we get a long list. But what we *should* be asking is, 'What beliefs need to be changed in order to make this person well?' And then the list will be shorter because once they find the healer, they may be ready to heal. But it all depends on being able to figure things out in the client–practitioner interaction. If the client is sick, the first thing to do is a healing and see if they get better.

I had a client with cancer throughout her body who'd had several chemo procedures. She was pushy and bold. I recognized her as a good healer and asked her, 'What have you done to fix this cancer?' She went off on a long list of the different things she had done. As she talked, I went up and asked, 'God, what does she need?'

I was told that she needed a little belief work. When I attempted a regular healing on her, the energy fell out of her body and had no effect. This response told me she had a broken heart, so I gave her the heart-song exercise (which I share in *Advanced ThetaHealing*) and told her to do it before working together again. There was change in her after that. I was expecting a long list, but it was a broken heart at the bottom of it.

—

Find out why and when the illness was created.

—

The digging work

Use the following process to uncover the key belief:

1. Find out why and when the illness was created.

2. Find out what the issues are and then start digging deeper by using the first two digging approaches.

3. Ask the client when the sickness started. If the client doesn't know, go up and ask the Creator for inspiration.

4. Ask what was going on in their life when the sickness began. Then dig deeper to resolve the issue.

Ask the following questions to uncover why the illness was created and why the person became sick.

- When did you first get sick?

- When did the illness start?

- What was going on in your life when you became sick?

Example

A good example of how a disease can bring positive aspects into someone's life is demonstrated in the following story.

A woman was walking down the road and was hit by a bus, which left her with broken bones that required surgery. When they cut her open, they found out that she had cancer. Now with broken bones, she began treatment for cancer, but nothing was working. After she was discharged from the hospital, she worked with many other ThetaHealers, as well as other modalities, before coming to see me. The doctors had given up on her and she sat in front of me saying, 'No one can help me.

What do I do?'

In this situation, I like to find out what was happening when the sickness first started.

Vianna: 'When did you first get cancer?'

Woman: *'I don't know when I got cancer.'*

(When I asked God, I was told that she had had it for seven years.)

Vianna: 'What happened seven years ago?'

When I first asked what was going on seven years ago, she couldn't remember. At first, she said everything was great at that time. This is where you should tell the client to go home and reflect upon everything that was going on in their life when the sickness started. She went home, found her journal and wrote everything down that was going on in her life at that time.

The next day we talked again. She told me that seven years ago she was still married, and her husband brought his mother home, who required a lot of care. The mother was very mean to her, so she went to her husband and gave him an ultimatum of 'It's either me or your mother.' This is generally a bad idea, since who did he pick? That's right, his mother. So, she told her husband, 'I'm going to leave you' and she left. So now her marriage had ended, and her children were angry with her. After spending all of her adult life with her husband and children, she had no financial (or emotional) support other than herself.

> **Vianna:** 'What has happened that is good in your life since the cancer?'

> **Woman:** *'When my husband and children found out I had cancer, I got back together with my husband and my relationship with my children was restored. Even my mother-in-law talked to me and treated me civilly.'*

Do you think she is going to give up the cancer that may have been created due to the stress of her mother-in-law moving in and the lack of love from her husband and children? She had lost everything and now because of the cancer her life was returned to her.

> **Vianna:** 'Is your husband going to stay with you if you recover from cancer?'

> **Woman:** *'No, he won't.'*

The real issues hadn't been addressed so she was going to stay sick as long as possible, so I started to do belief work on:

'I am lovable.'

'I can be loved without being sick.'

'I can be strong without being sick.'

'My family will love me without me being sick.'

We didn't work on the cancer itself but that she could be loved without the cancer. After we worked on these issues, we did a healing on the cancer. After two or three weeks, she called me to say that the cancer had gone into remission.

The belief work I did with her wasn't specifically on the cancer itself but on the following programs:

'I am lovable without being sick.'

'My husband will stay with me if I am sick.'

'I must be sick to stay with my family.'

DIGGING APPROACH 4: ILLNESS 2

Find out how the illness is serving the client. Ask the client to go into the future and ask them what would happen if the sickness was gone and they got better? How would they deal with this new situation?

An example of this is a client that had diabetes. I asked him how he would deal with being completely well in the future. I asked this because I knew the diabetes had started when he was a teenager, so he would be able to remember what it felt like to feel healthy.

He told me that if he didn't have diabetes he would become more physically active and move away from the city to be with his friends. As he imagined this future, his face changed and took on the energy of health before changing to a look of horror.

He said, 'If I become healthy, my wife will leave me because she doesn't like my friends and dislikes the outdoors. She loves city life and my diabetes is the only thing we have in common. She helps me take care of it. If I am well she will leave me, or I will leave her.'

Then I asked him if he wanted to change a few things to be able to share his interests and love of nature with his wife. But instead of being open to change, he refused and ended the session.

Sometimes people are more afraid of becoming well than of being sick. For example, they may be afraid they will lose their medical benefits and have to work again. Find out the client's true motivation behind their illness. Change this belief so that the client is motivated to become completely well.

Start the digging work

To find out why someone is sick, ask:

- What is going to happen to you if you get better?

- What would happen if you were completely healed?

- How has the illness served you, and what did you get out of it that is positive?

- What was the best thing that happened to you from being sick?

- What did you learn from being sick?

But how can someone get healthy if their focus isn't on getting well?

The following exchange with a man who came to see me with HIV serves as a good example.

> **Vianna:** 'OK, you have HIV. What is going to happen if you get better?'
>
> **Man:** 'Oh, I don't want to get better. I just want you to lower my viral load. I don't want it to go away, because if it goes away I will lose my father and my family.'
>
> **Vianna:** 'What?'

Man: *'My father hated that I was homosexual and disowned me. But now I have HIV, he is in my life again. I eat better, I take better care of myself and I have a family again.'*

Vianna: 'Would like to know you can have all that without the HIV?'

Man: *'No, I don't want to be well. I only want to lower my viral load, so it doesn't turn into AIDS.'*

Vianna: 'Wouldn't you like to know your father could love you without you being sick?'

Man: *'No, I know my father. This is all I want.'*

This exchange told me why he was holding on to the HIV. His father's love was more important. So, I did what he asked and did a healing on his viral load.

When I ask clients, 'What good thing has happened to you since you developed breast cancer,' most will say 'My family has come together.' These positive energies hold on to the disease. This is because we are sparks of God. We create things for a purpose.

The short and the long list

Each person has a long list of things to do to heal. A long list can be overwhelming, so it is best to start with the short list. The long list pertains to their whole life on all levels and the short list is focused on the illness. First heal the short-term issues and then work on their long-term health and neither you nor the client become overwhelmed.

It is also worth noting that some healers attempt to *make* their clients live because they are attached to them. If the client becomes better, you will still be attached to them. If the client goes to another dimension, you will still be attached to them. And remember not everyone that is sick is also pleasant. Mean people get sick too.

If you think your client is sick and they need you, remember they are sick and need the Creator. You are the witness. The pressure of feeling that you are a client's last hope can be difficult to deal with. You may end up feeling emotionally involved and pleading to God; 'Please God, please God, help this person.'

DIGGING APPROACH 5: MANIFESTING

This approach uses digging to free the client's mind so that they can manifest their dreams. Digging to create manifestation is focusing on what will happen in the future once the client has what they want. This means telling the client to imagine what it would be like to have what they want.

Manifesting for abundance isn't simply about asking for material wealth, because the universe knows that money is made of paper and so does the subconscious. Instead manifest for what you would *do* with the money and then let the universe fill in the blanks.

The goals list

If we don't create a list of goals every year to maintain the soul's focus, we can manifest the weirdest problems to keep us entertained – because without challenges we get bored. I have observed this in many of my students, as well as myself. If we aren't manifesting in all avenues of our lives, the universe will fill in the blanks for us.

This is why giving the universe a continual list of manifestations that work for you instead of against you is so important. If you say, 'Everything is perfect in my life, I don't want anything,' the universe will create something for you – and it may be something you don't want. For example, if you want a new crystal you might manifest, 'I need $15,000 to buy a new crystal.' However, it is *the crystal you need*, not the money, and so that is what you manifest for. That way when someone gives you a crystal – because it is taking too much room in their house and they know you would appreciate it – it is incidental that the crystal is worth $15. You would be surprised at how often this happens.

The problem with manifesting for only one thing at a time is that healers are very intuitive, and if they have a list then the subconscious will treat it like a 'grocery list' and check off the topics one by one and make them happen. If the only thing you give your subconscious to work on is financial security, it can take a lifetime for it to complete this one goal. So, it is better to manifest for at least 10 things at once.

Being in sync with divine timing

Many years ago, I wasn't manifesting as I should, so I decided to manifest something so that the universe didn't fill in the blanks. I decided I wanted a place where I could raise organic vegetables for my classes and went up and manifested 10 acres of land and within a week my husband's father gave us a 250-acre farm. This was a little overwhelming at first because the place needed quite a lot of fixing up and so it took some time before I could start raising organic vegetables!

I asked myself, 'So now I have a farm what am I going to do with it?' Initially the farm was used as a wintering ground for cows, but I wasn't good with cows, so I decided to raise horses.

I had wanted to raise Friesian horses since seeing the movie *Lady and the Hawk* – the Friesian black horse in the movie was so stately and gentle. The Friesian line comes from the Netherlands and was originally bred to carry knights into battle. But as the need for a knightly horse went out of vogue they were used for dressage and drawing carriages and light draft. My desire to own a Friesian horse was somewhat unfocused: I knew I wanted one, but this desire wasn't yet connected to the rest of my life. However, I did know that I was more suited to looking at horses than actually taking care of them and knew I would need someone to take care of it for me. So I went online to buy a Friesian mare and, when I found one I liked, I asked the Creator about it and was told 'If this horse stays where it is it will die."

With any conversation with the Creator, it is always best to ask a broad range of questions, such as 'Can I save this horse or is it going to die anyway?' But I didn't ask this important question and purchased the horse, so I could save her. I shipped the mare to the farm from California and about two weeks later she died. When I got my daughter's message, her tone scared me at first, because she was acting like someone in the family had died. Her news made me sad, but I was very relieved to find out that it was the horse and not one of my children.

I asked, 'God, why did this horse die?'

God said, 'Vianna, you didn't listen to the message. You buy a dead horse, you get a dead horse. The grain she was given in California made her sick.' (I wouldn't have had this lesson if I had listened to what I was being told.)

The veterinarian came and tested the mare to find the cause of death and, sure enough, traces of ergot (moldy grain) showed up in her tissues. This type of mold is a problem in California and was likely due to moisture getting into the grain storage unit. This type of mold is deadly to a pregnant horse and it was the veterinarian's opinion that she had been fed poisoned feed for a while.

The insurance covered the cost of the horse and, undeterred but much wiser, I decided to manifest the same desire again under a much stricter criterion. Since I'd lost a horse I decided to manifest two horses and found two Friesians from Carolina. But this time I manifested under the auspices of ThetaHealing as representations for the animal class I teach. This means there had to be a direct correlation between the horses and ThetaHealing in order for it to work for me. The other change I made was to raise high-ranking Friesian horses to help save the breed.

This is also why it is very important to know your **divine timing** and to interconnect manifestations with it, not against it. If your divine timing is to influence a million people and you manifest wanting to live alone on a desert island, you more than likely won't get it. But if the desert island will be used for influencing those million people then you may well manifest your desire.

—

You can manifest anything, as long as it is in sync with your divine timing.

—

Soul mates and healing centers

When manifesting, imagine what it feels like to have your desire and once you receive the manifestation, take responsibility for it. In other words, if you buy a horse, you have to take care of it and if you manifest for a soul mate you will have to live with them.

Often people say they want to manifest a soul mate but what they actually *want* is a *compatible* soul mate. After all, most of us don't want a mate we can simply order around and take out of the closet when we need them. We want someone with a brain and that isn't easy – and healers, in particular, never want things to be easy. However, sometimes it is better to manifest for a compatible soul mate until you are ready to allow them to be a divine life partner. And if you want a divine life partner, you need first to ask *if* the person is ready for you and *if* you are ready for them. I dreamed about Guy for 10 years before I met him. If I had met him any sooner, we wouldn't have got along so well. It only worked because we were both ready to meet each other.

Put simply, understand that when you make a manifestation you might just get it. If your subconscious feels that receiving the manifestation will bring too much danger, too much stress or is simply too much for you, it will stop the manifesting from happening. This is also why it is important to work through the possibilities of why your subconscious might block the manifestation.

Always ask, 'What is going to happen if I get the manifestation?'

For example, many healers want to manifest a healing center. When I hear this, I usually say, 'Are you crazy? Do you really want to work in a healing center with other healers?'

After all, a healing center sounds like the ideal environment, but the mix of healers' personalities can feel very different in reality – and competition is always a factor. So, if manifesting a healing center is on your list, I also recommend manifesting healers that have morals, integrity, and can work together, as well as a good accountant.

Perhaps you want to manifest being a successful healer, but do you really want this? Think about what would happen if you did six appointments in a day and every one of your clients healed? The next day you would have 50 phone calls. Then what if every one of those 50 people healed as well? By the end of the week, you might have 1,000 people asking for healings. What would happen if you had 1,000 people asking for healings? And if somehow you were able to heal those people, 10,000 would be after you for healings – weeping and sick and screaming for healings. At some point, being a successful healer will become overwhelming, which is why healers only want a few people to get better at a time.

And if your clients aren't getting better, you have to learn to be a better healer. In order to be a better healer, know that God is the healer and find the client's belief, but also know that you can't make anyone heal if they don't want to. It is important to tell your clients that you can work with them, but the Creator is the healer.

In order to manifest being a better healer, release any fears, doubts, and disbeliefs associated with it. Understand that you have to be kind, considerate, and non-judgmental. If you manifest being a better healer and don't have the right abilities, the universe will bring you situations to teach you them, because all manifestations have consequences associated with them.

Start the digging work

Ask the client to visualize what they would do with their life if they had plenty of money – more than they could ever spend. Then ask the client to elaborate on the situation by asking the following questions while they visualize the outcome:

- Where are you?

- How do you feel?

- Who is with you?

- How do your family/friends/soul mate react to this abundance?

Continue the digging work

Discover the issues that make the client feel uncomfortable in their visualization and start digging deeper to resolve any issues which may be blocking them from creating abundance.

Ask questions to identify the issues and encourage the client to visualize having all the abundance they ever wanted. Ask the client to visualize:

- What would you do if you had all the money you ever wanted?

- Where would you be if you had all the money you ever wanted?

- How do you feel with all the money you ever wanted?

- Where would you live?

- Who is with you? What do they look like?

- Is there a significant other in your life and if there is, how do your family and friends react to all that money?

- How do your family and friends react to your manifestation?

- What person or people in your life would be upset with you if you were successful?

- What would they say to you?

- What could go wrong if you have everything you want?

- What is the best thing that would happen if you had everything you wanted?

DIGGING APPROACH 6: GENETICS

When energy testing for beliefs, there will be times when the client has no conscious awareness of some of the programs that come up. When this happens, the client may become confused, making it difficult to continue the digging work. This scenario is likely to happen when the beliefs are genetic in nature – passed down through the DNA from their ancestors. (*See also page 40.*) For example, the client may have prejudice, anger, or resentment against certain people. The ancestor's beliefs may also be outdated and not serving them in their current lifetime.

Ancestors

If you can't find the answers to where the belief comes from then it is time to look at the client's ancestors, and ask:

- What were they like?

- What did they believe and how much did their beliefs affect them?

- What kinds of energies did they inherit from them?

I once took over an intuitive anatomy class that my son was teaching (because of an emergency). There were only 10 students and I hadn't taught such a small class for many years, let alone a basic class. You see, the smaller the class, the more questions people will ask. While this is OK, it also means students can take you off task and gives them an opportunity to grandstand – as well as other display behaviors that aren't conducive to a learning environment.

It was time to do a demonstration of belief work and one of the students, a young British man, a 21-year-old Capricorn, seemed to think that he knew *everything* and refused to do any belief work because he thought that he was perfect. After the first week and having worked with him in belief-work sessions, the rest of the students were becoming increasingly frustrated with him.

While he was quick to point out the flaws in others, (he thought) he had none himself. The other students knew that he had a lot of issues, but he wouldn't work on any of them. It became apparent that in order to save him from the rest of the class (who were plotting a British barbecue), I should bring him up and work with him in front of the class:

Vianna: 'Let's do some belief work.'

Student: *'I am perfectly fine, everything is going perfectly fine in my life and I don't need belief work.'*

Vianna: 'OK, so let's work on your father instead and then you will be able to tell if you have inherited any genetic programs from him – but of course, you have only inherited them, you don't actually *have* them. If we can change them in you, they can change in him, if he accepts it.'

(He became very animated at that point.)

Student: *'I would love to work on that.'*

Vianna: 'OK, what would you like to work on?'

Student: *'My father, you can't tell him anything! He knows everything. He never listens to anyone else; he thinks he is perfect and doesn't listen to anything I say. He wants me to be a lawyer, but I want to be a musician and it is impossible to communicate with him. I would like to change this about my father.'*

(At this point the other students raised their eyebrows.)

Vianna: 'Why do you think that your father is like this?'

Student: *'He was older than my mother when they got married. My father was a prisoner of war and the only member of his platoon to survive capture. He learned the only person he could depend on in order to stay alive was himself.'*

Vianna: 'Would you like to know it is safe to listen to others' opinions and that you can make your own decisions? That it is safe to listen and safe to be alive?'

(After these downloads, he started working with others in the class.)

Later he called me and said, 'Vianna, that work we did in class really worked! My father listens to me and is letting me go back to school to be a musician instead of a lawyer. Thank you for changing my life.'

This is a good example of how ancestral programs can affect our lives and how there is always something for us to work on.

Start the digging work

The way to begin ancestral work is to start with the client's parents. The best way to look at our parents is with some compassion because they were not taught how to be parents.

Ask questions:

- What is your family like?

- What do they believe?

- Where did they come from?

- What happened to your mother, your father, or their parents?

In some instances, the client won't have direct knowledge about their ancestors and this is where your intuition comes in. You are going to have to ask the client to touch their skin and look inwardly to see what comes up in the way of beliefs.

Every time you do deep-level digging work, your client will change on a genetic level – sometimes even in their genetic predisposition. Obviously genetic tendencies are now well established in medicine, but recent scientific testing strongly suggests that people who went through a traumatic experience may have also sent trauma down to their children and their children and so on.

The research, led by Rachel Yehuda, stems from the genetic study of 32 Jewish men and women who were either interned in a Nazi concentration camp, witnessed or experienced torture, or had to hide during World War II. The researchers also analyzed the genes of their children, who are known to have an increased likelihood of stress disorders compared to Jewish families who lived outside Europe during the war. 'The gene changes in the children could only be attributed to Holocaust exposure in the parents,' said Yehuda.[3]

Her team's work is the clearest example in humans of the transmission of trauma to a child via what is called 'epigenetic inheritance' – the idea that environmental influences such as smoking, diet, and stress can affect the genes of children and possibly even grandchildren.

The study of epigenetics is still controversial because scientific convention states that genes contained in DNA are the only way to transmit biological information between generations. However, our genes are modified by the environment all the time through chemical tags which attach themselves to our DNA and switch genes on and off. Recent studies suggest that some of these tags might somehow be passed through generations – meaning our environment could also have an impact on our children's health.

Researchers were specifically interested in one region of a gene associated with the regulation of stress hormones, which is known to be affected by trauma.[4] 'It makes sense to look at this gene,' said Yehuda. 'If there's a transmitted effect of trauma, it would be in a stress-related gene that shapes the way we cope with our environment.'[3]

Continue the digging work

If the client says it is wrong to heal themselves, it is probably an ancestral belief. Past oaths, vows, or commitments – such as being humble and poor to be closer to the Creator – are almost always no longer useful in modern life and should be changed in order to help the client heal.

Example

Practitioner: 'Why can't you heal?'

Client: *'It is wrong for me to heal myself, because healing means I am being selfish.'*

Ask the following questions and continue digging to identify the genetic issue by asking the client if a certain belief is the client's mother's, father's, or an ancestor's.

- Is this your mother's belief?

- Is this your father's belief?

- Is this your ancestor's belief?

- If you could work on your father or mother, what belief would you want to work on?

- How did it serve them and what did they get out of it?

- Have they learned everything that it needed to teach them?

If the client energy tests with a 'Yes' response, download the client that 'it is completed' and the feeling that they can move forward.

—

Remember not all ancestral beliefs need to be changed because many – such as stubbornness, humor, and perseverance, for example – are beneficial.

—

DIGGING APPROACH 7: HISTORY LEVEL

When we learn to go into a Theta state, our psychic senses open and we may also experience past-life remembrances. As a practitioner, this is something to be aware of so that you can guide the client through this delicate time. If the client becomes so consumed with memories, it will make it difficult for them to understand what really matters and move forward.

This is why, when history-level beliefs come up in a digging session, you need to energy test the client to check that the past life is *complete*. If you receive a 'Yes' response, you can download that these problems are completed. If they energy test with a 'No' response then you should ask the client what they have learned from their past life.

Generally, only one-tenth of clients will need to work on this level. In fact, most of the people who come to ThetaHealing classes have already graduated from the energy of the Third Plane and their past lives are resolved, but this doesn't keep them from remembering them.

In dealing with history-level beliefs, the first-remembered past lives are also usually the most tragic. In readings, you'll find that people always talk about their hardships first and getting stuck in a past life can cause a real problem in belief work. It is easy to become consumed with past-life energies, unless we take the good from those experiences and go on with life. Our focus should be to help this planet wake up in the here and now.

—

If it helps to remember another time and place that's good, but many a good psychic gets caught up in the past.

—

I was 31 when I had my second major past-life experience during some **release work**. It was such a strong memory that the massage table I was lying on broke – just snapped in two for no reason. The memory was so detailed: I was an Egyptian high priestess and they had cut out my heart. I became consumed with the remembrance of this time and spent a year attempting to remember more and resolve problems. I now appreciate that I was lucky not to become completely consumed by it.

At first, what I remembered from my first past-life experience was that the people that love you betray you. But when I asked God about the lifetime I was told: 'You need to change that belief and no, that isn't what you learned.' Then the Creator showed me the virtues I had learned in that lifetime; it was one of the two lifetimes from which I gained many of the virtues that I carry from life to life.

Other psychics I know weren't so fortunate. For example, one psychic I know remembered she was Chief Red Cloud in a past life. She was so consumed with this memory that it affected her mental stability and she ended up in jail telling people that she was Chief Red Cloud. Remember, there are many reasons for past-life memories; they could come from genetics or from other influences.

Some people accumulate these essences and carry beliefs from past lives, such as a **vow** of poverty. As a practitioner, you can just go up and command that it is simply gone. However, on some level, the oath was taken for a reason and attempting to erase it will do no good since it will reinstall itself. But if you recognize that the past-life experience was viable then the energy of the oath can be transformed or shifted into the present life as *completed*. Then you can energy test the client to see if the oath or vow is completed. If there is something that the client remembers with clarity, you can ask them what they learned from that lifetime.

Sometimes psychics use past lives as a screen to avoid dealing with the underlying problem. When a client starts talking about past lives, some healers will use the excuse of 'I will be killed for being a healer' to move forward as a healer. This is true of most healers in the past and can make us more afraid of success and publicity than we are of failure. But this is also why we should seek to resolve these programs – because it is our mission, the reason we came here.

In every lifetime, we achieve different virtues; however, there are generally two or three lifetimes where we achieve more virtues than others. These are the ones that we remember the most and I call them 'graduating lifetimes.' As masters in this existence we are attempting to remember all the virtues that we have achieved and mastered, remembering that virtues are the highest thought vibrations. I list the virtues that are needed to be a good healer in *Planes of Existence*.

Past-life beliefs

In reality, we all have the birthright to ask the Creator for healings. But if we have certain virtues, the healings will be more consistent. One of the virtues needed for healing is kindness. When the master remembers the virtue of kindness, the lifetime in which someone has mastered the virtue of kindness will come to mind.

As I described earlier in the book, there are four levels where beliefs are held in an individual:

- Core

- Genetic

- History

- Soul

Some of the beliefs inherent on the history level include past-life beliefs and group-conscious beliefs.

The history level has energetic memories which make us what we are and help us to grow. However, some of these experiences may be negative in nature and these energies need to be resolved. In this case, you will need to witness the client's trauma and drama and resolve these emotional energies by sending them to God's light – while also helping the client to see any learnings from the memory.

For instance, let's say someone was burnt at the stake for being a healer in a past life. In the present time, they are being attacked for being a healer since they are somehow unconsciously recreating the situation. This means that they need to resolve the past-life issue by sending away the pain and anguish of that experience. In this way they don't keep reliving the event but keep the memory of being a healer.

A good example of a belief from the history level is one I mentioned earlier in the book: the student who thought she was Joan of Arc (*see page 69*). During digging the student said, 'I must sacrifice my life for my beliefs,' and believed she was Joan of Arc. Whether it was 'true' or where it came from doesn't really matter. What mattered was changing the belief that she must die for what she believes, and the energy of the belief is completed. Then she was able to believe what she needed to, but still lead a healthy life.

—

We don't attempt to pull the belief of who the client believes they were, but rather replace the residual belief that is causing a problem.

—

The presence of past-life beliefs doesn't necessarily mean they were actually lived. Some intuitive people accumulate the memories of another individual's past life from ghost imprints or inanimate objects such as crystals. The old memories of these imprints can be confused for past lives. Everything we touch leaves our essence on it, as does anything touched by others. Some of these energies can come from genetic memories or from the Akashic records. When we are in the right state of mind, we can experience some of these overlapping memories.

Group conscious beliefs

When many people have the same belief, such as 'diabetes is incurable,' they accept it as a fact and it becomes a group conscious belief. When enough people believe the same thing, it becomes part of the collective consciousness of humankind. Once an intuitive person connects to the collective consciousness, it can be accepted and confused with an ultimate truth. When this happens, the belief needs to be changed to a positive energy.

Examples of group conscious beliefs include:

'Diabetes is incurable.'

'The end of the world is coming.'

'It was my fault that Atlantis was destroyed.'

'I am afraid of using my power.'

'I took a vow of poverty.'

Start the digging work

Find these beliefs and change them, so that the beliefs don't affect the client's life. Make the command or request: 'This is completed now. This is finished. I am ready to move forward. Thank you. It is done. It is done. It is done.'

Continue the belief work by asking:

- When did it start?

- What did you get out of this?

- What did you learn from it?

- Is it completed? If the answer is 'Yes,' command that 'it is completed in this life' and 'I no longer need it.'

DIGGING APPROACH 8: THE IMPOSSIBLE

Even though the Creator is doing the healing, you are the witness. If you believe that the healing is impossible, the witnessing of the healing will also be impossible. In fact, anytime that you think that it is impossible to heal something, of course it is impossible! That is why we are ThetaHealers, because we are really good at doing the impossible. Our job is 'everything is possible.'

Some scientists believe that many things are impossible, including healing. And yet, conventional medicine has only just discovered a hitherto-unknown organ in the body – termed the 'interstitium'; one that was missed in the last 150 years of anatomical study and may help medical researchers to understand how cancer spreads.[5] Similarly, scientists used to think the pineal gland had no purpose and, when I was little, doctors arbitrarily removed tonsils on the pretext that they were 'useless.'

When I lived in Idaho I went to the doctor because I wasn't feeling well. During the physical exam, the doctor looked in my throat and told me I had the biggest tonsils she had ever seen, and asked why they hadn't been removed long before? This didn't feel right to me and I refused to have surgery and did a healing on it instead. It was about this time that I also moved from Idaho to Montana.

When I lived in Idaho I was allergic to every bush and shrub (according to the doctor). However, when I moved to Montana and went to a doctor for the same allergy tests, I wasn't allergic to anything. But you know what else was gone? My swollen tonsils. This doctor told me that he couldn't find my tonsils and asked me if I'd had them removed. Yet the other doctor, a year before, told me that I had the biggest tonsils she had ever seen. That must be impossible!

I put the allergy medical record with all the others, like the congestive heart failure (when I survived the doctor said, 'Oh, not really.'), the tumor in my leg (to which the doctors said, 'I don't know where it went.'). All these records are in a safe so that one day someone will look at them and see they were all impossible.

—

Impossible is brain candy.

—

I once worked with a little girl age three with diabetes type 1. I did a healing on her and witnessed the Creator work on her

DNA. Since the healing, the child hadn't used insulin for five years, but the child's mother said, 'My daughter has diabetes type 1 and it has been five years since she's used insulin.' In stating her daughter 'has diabetes type 1,' she is hopeful the diabetes has gone but doesn't really believe it. Somewhere in her subconscious, she believed the diabetes was still there.

Intuitive healing is also related to how much we have cleared beliefs pertaining to what is perceived as impossible. Belief work should be focused on what is perceived as impossible to become possible. In the DNA 3 class, ThetaHealers learn to do healing work on their environment and the planet by becoming aware of the impossible beliefs inherent in massive group-consciousness beliefs. They begin to learn who they are, not as a three-dimensional being, but as multidimensional being having a three-dimensional experience. This human body is our life-support system, but we are more than the physical. Proving this involves convincing students that they *can* move matter with pure thought. But many students give up on these exercises because they believe they are impossible. Impossible things can be done.

Start the digging work

When faced with changing beliefs of the impossible some people think that they will leave their families and move on to another dimension. These are real fears and the client may need a lot of downloads to make them feel comfortable.

In belief work, the questions to ask are:

- What's going to happen if you can do what you think is impossible?

- What is going to happen if you can move matter with your mind?

- What's going to happen if you can witness healings?

These questions are some things that can bring up terrible fears in people such as:

'If I can do this people will be afraid of me.'

'People will try to kill me.'

'Only Christ can heal.'

'It's wrong to be like Christ.'

'If I do "magic" I can be burned as a witch.'

Clients often believe that changing beliefs about the impossible is difficult and so it is important to clear these and other fears, so the client understands that it is safe to do so, and they won't misuse their abilities as a result.

The New Testament tells us that Christ did many miracles. In essence Christ said, 'You can do the things that I can do.' But there was another man named Apollonius who, at the same time, was purported to have done healings much the same as Christ, however, very little was written about him. There have been numerous references throughout history about miraculous healings. At some point in the development of Christianity, healers were either made into saints or burned at the stake – depending on the attitude at the time.

In some group consciousness, it is believed healing someone with the energy of thought and prayer is impossible. From this, we learn that the fears, doubts, and disbeliefs of others will accomplish nothing. Unlike the other digging methods that are used to find blocks, this digging method is used to reprogram the brain to accept that the impossible can be changed with the power of focused thought and prayer.

In this exploration, we learn to work on what the individual's subconscious thinks is impossible; to teach them that it is beliefs in the mind that keep this reality in place. In this way, what seems impossible may actually become possible. On every level, you were taught that this was impossible, but it is wrong somehow.

The first thing to teach yourself is that something is possible. The issues that can come up in belief work with a client are fears such as 'people will think that I am different,' 'people will try to hurt me,' or 'if I am different I won't fit in,' for example. So, you might have to use fear work (the first digging approach) in order to clear issues about the impossible.

—

It is important to develop the ability to use any of the 10 digging approaches in a session as the need presents itself.

—

Continue the digging work

If the client expresses programs and beliefs about what they believe is impossible in the digging process, it is useful to change these beliefs, so they can accept a healing.

Tell the client to avoid the use of the following expressions, either in their spoken statements or thoughts.

'I can't...'

'My problem is...'

'That is impossible...'

'Yes, but it doesn't work for me.'

Ask the client the following questions:

- What would happen if...?

- What would happen if you could do this?

- Why is it impossible?

- Who told you that it was impossible?

Download the belief of the 'impossible is completed' and 'it is possible.'

DIGGING APPROACH 9: PRESENT DIGGING – LEARNING FROM HARDSHIPS

In this digging approach, you guide the client to state their present problem and then ask what they are getting out of it, 'What benefit are you getting from the hardships that you are experiencing?'

For every hardship there is a deeper reason for it happening. Our soul is learning from every life experience. It doesn't matter to the soul if these are good or bad experiences, but it does matter what we acquire from them. If we can learn virtues through a difficult situation then this is a good thing for the soul and why it is important to recognize the good things that we have learned from any hardships. In this way we won't have to repeat the hardships in other situations and can develop spiritually without them.

Start the digging work

In this digging approach, you guide the client to state the problem they are experiencing in the present time. Then you ask the client what they are learning from it.

The following belief-work session is a good example:

In the session, the man told me he had moved his mother into his house and she was driving him crazy. I asked him, 'What are you getting out of having your mother in your house?'

He thought for a while before replying, 'My mother was a very controlling person when I was younger. She controlled everything in my life. Now that she is in my life I control everything in her life. My brothers and sister won't come and see me anymore because they dislike her, so now they can't ask me for a loan.'

Suddenly, he saw the situation he had created on a deep subconscious level and how it was serving him.

I taught him to understand his mother, so he could live with her. I also taught him how to live without having to control her. The man was able to live a more harmonious life as a result.

—

**There is much that can be changed
by working on ourselves.**

—

In another case, a woman came to me for a reading.

Woman: 'For some reason I can't make any more money than what I am currently making. I am blocked for some reason. I am in a divorce and I am suffering so much.'

Vianna: 'OK, *close your eyes and tell me, what are you getting out of suffering so much?*'

Woman: 'I don't get anything out of this. I am struggling.'

Vianna: 'OK *close your eyes and go up and ask the Creator, 'What am I getting out of this struggling?'*'

(She closed her eyes for a few moments before speaking.)

Woman: 'As long as I only make so much money I don't have to give my husband half. When we are divorced I can keep all the money I make.'

This realization was life changing for her. She just had to understand why it was so difficult. And when the divorce was complete, she started to make plenty of money.

In another session, a client was seeking a soul mate and asked me to help her.

Woman: 'Why can't I find my soul mate? I have looked and looked for 10 years. I have done everything. Why can't I find him?'

Vianna: *'What are you getting out of not having a soul mate?'*

Woman: 'Nothing, I want one!'

Vianna: *'Close your eyes and think. What do you get out of this?'*

(She thought about it before speaking.)

Woman: 'As long as I am looking for a soul mate I don't have to have one. I like my house. I like the way I live but everyone thinks I should have a soul mate. But if I get a soul mate, he will change the way I live and the way I am. I don't want to change.'

In 30 seconds, she had received the answer to why she wasn't getting what she thought she wanted.

In conversation, a friend told me, 'I can't drop this weight,' while munching on a chocolate bar.

I asked her, 'What do you get out of being fat?'

She looked at me and said, 'You know I am an older woman. If I drop weight I will become wrinkled. I don't want to be wrinkled. If I drop weight my husband becomes more jealous and I don't want to be a shriveled prune.'

—

Belief work on hardships will always show the hidden motivations that we try to avoid seeing.

—

This woman came to me because she had nearly divorced 14 times; her husband left her at the same time every year.

Vianna: 'Your husband leaves you at the same time every year?'

Client: *'Yes.'*

Vianna: 'And does he come back?'

Client: *'Yes.'*

Vianna: 'How does this happen? Does he pack up all his things and leave?'

Client: *'Yes. He tells me that we should divorce, and I should change my name and it is forever. He starts to sell our house and then returns and says, "We are married again."'*

Vianna: 'Close your eyes and tell me, what do you get out of that situation?'

Client: *'The first time it happened, I was sick and returned to healing work. First, I did psychotherapy and then I started ThetaHealing. I opened a new center and began traveling. When he decided to leave me, I was traveling, making new projects and was very happy. When he decided to return I felt heavy at first,* but then I realized that together we have better possibilities in life. I realized that we love each other. Still two parts of myself are fighting each other in the marriage. One part wants to be free and the other wants to be married. Then the cycle starts over again, and things become difficult between us.'

Vianna: 'OK, when he leaves you can play a little bit and it is easier to do your healing. Do you date when he is gone?'

Client: 'No, I don't want someone else. When he is gone he is jealous of me but feels better than when he's with me.

Vianna: 'So, you kind of like him to do this. It gives you freedom, helps you to accomplish other projects, and then you get your marriage back.'

Client: 'When we get back together it is on a new level and different every time.'

Vianna: 'As long as you are ready to get divorced, you don't have to get divorced and you keep some of your freedom.'

Client: 'Yes, and I don't need a new man in my life.'

Vianna: 'This sounds like it keeps your relationship very interesting.'

Client: 'But now we are tired of the situation.'

Vianna: 'Let's see. I'm going to energy test you. Repeat after me: "I am tired of my husband leaving and coming back."'

Client: 'I am tired of my husband leaving me and coming back.'

(She energy tests with a 'No' response.)

Vianna: 'Say, "I enjoy having a break from my husband."'

Client: *'I enjoy having a break from my husband.'*

(She energy tests with a 'Yes' response.)

Vianna: 'Say, "My family is tired of this situation."'

Client: *'My family is tired of this situation.'*

(She energy tests with a 'Yes' response.)

Vianna: 'My father and mother are tired of the situation.'

Client: *'They don't know about it.'*

Vianna: 'OK, who else knows about it?'

Client: *'My children are tired of the situation.'*

(She energy tests with a 'Yes' response.)

Vianna: 'Say, "I like the situation."'

Client: *'I like the situation.'*

(She energy tests with a 'Yes' response.)

Vianna: Say, "As long as this situation continues, my husband and I can keep starting over and over again."'

Client: *'As long as this situation continues my husband and I can keep starting over and over again.'*

(She energy tests with a 'Yes' response.)

Vianna: 'Would you like to know that you can still have some of your freedom without this situation, and you can start over without breaking up and coming back together?'

Client: *'Yes.'*

Vianna: 'Say, "I get bored being married."'

Client: *'I get bored being married.'*

(She energy tests with a 'Yes' response.)

Vianna: 'Would you like to know that you can create excitement in your marriage?'

Client: *'Yes, I get bored.'*

Vianna: 'Can we change your fear of being bored?'

Client: *'Yes.'*

Vianna: 'Can I change the belief of "I am bored" to "marriage can be exciting"?'

Client: *'Yes. When I chose a husband, I made sure he was difficult. All the men I dated that were positive were also boring.'*

As you can see we found what she was getting out of the situation and there were a lot of positive things. Then we taught her that she could have positive things without creating that situation. Then we energy tested her to see if that situation was over.

> **Vianna:** 'Say, "I need to create this situation with my husband."'

> **Client:** *'I need to create this situation with my husband.'*

(She energy tests with a 'Yes' response.)

> **Vianna:** 'So, when do you think you will stop creating this situation? A year? Two years?'

> **Client:** *'I can't understand why I need this situation.'*

> **Vianna:** 'Well, you get a chance to be free and create.'

> **Client:** *'When I am traveling and we are apart I feel guilty, but when he leaves I don't feel guilty. When I return home I am very kind.'*

> **Vianna:** 'Would you like to change that? Would you like to know that you can travel without feeling guilty and you can travel together?'

> **Client:** *'I want to travel without feeling guilty but when we travel together I have to pay for everything because he never has money.'*

Vianna: 'But you are married. Don't you share money?'

Client: *'I make most of the money in the relationship.'*

Vianna: 'Is it "your money" in the relationship?'

Client: *'Yes.'*

Vianna: 'But you love him. When you love someone it's OK to travel and share the money. Would you like to know that you can make so much money that you can travel together and have his company? And you can find an even balance in your relationship so that he feels important?'

Client: *'Yes, and that I will have enough for myself, for him and my children.'*

Vianna: 'Would you like to know how to share your money with the one you love without getting resentful, and that you are allowed to make more being together – knowing that he can help you be safe?'

Client: *'Yes.'*

Vianna: 'Say, "It's wrong for a woman to make more than a man."'

Client: *'It's wrong for a woman to make more than a man.'*

(She energy tests with a 'Yes' response.)

Vianna: 'This might be a genetic program. Would you like to know that it is amazing to make money and that you can make money without a sense of guilt and it can be accepted?'

We had found what she was getting out of the situation but as we kept digging we found more things to work on.

Vianna: 'What virtue did you learn from this situation?'

Client: *'I am learning forgiveness and to love him completely.'*

Vianna: 'Have you learned how to share? How to forgive him?'

Client: *'I learned how to feel him, and I learned clairvoyance because I can read his mind. I have learned how to respect his free will.'*

Vianna: 'You have also learned how to be a great healer and you can succeed by yourself. Would you like to know that you have learned from these things? And are you ready to learn more and know it is completed? And can you recognize these things?'

(The client is crying.)

Client: *'Yes.'*

Vianna: 'And would you like to know how to let him love you completely?'

Client: *'Yes.'*

Vianna: 'When you travel, it isn't that you mind sharing with him but that you feel used. Would you like to see the good parts of him when you travel?'

Client: *'Yes.'*

At the end of the session the client knew what she was getting out of the relationship and what she was learning from it.

Here are some questions you could ask yourself or a client to identify any issues of unnecessary hardship:

• Why are you permitting people to treat you as they do?

• Why do you have financial troubles?

• Why do you struggle with love?

• How is this hardship helping you?

• What are you getting out of it?

• Why did you create it?

• What virtue are you developing from the hardship?

• How can you develop virtues without hardships?

- Do you know what it feels like to live without hardships and still develop virtues?

DIGGING APPROACH 10: LEARNING VIRTUES

What are you learning from hardships and challenges? What virtues are you developing from your experiences?

The soul's purpose in this life is to learn virtues and develop abilities. As described earlier in the book, a virtue is a lite thought form that permits us to create. These virtuous thoughts free us from the materialistic anchor of the body. Non-virtuous thoughts are heavy and block our inherent abilities. For instance, if you want to be a better healer, you need the virtues of kindness, non-judgment, and caring for others. We are given opportunities to develop virtues throughout our lives; the trick is to develop them without having to experience difficult situations first.

The soul has to develop virtues to be able to achieve its divine timing (required for manifestation, as described above). This means that everything we have ever done matters. Every experience good or bad matters as it has taught us something good.

But what abilities do we need? If we ask the Creator how to be a better healer, then every fear, doubt, and disbelief about healing may come up. But to be better healers we have to be kind, tolerant, patient, caring, and have the ability to interact with other people without judgment.

As soon as we become aware of these virtues, the soul starts to work to achieve them. This gives us the opportunity of working toward virtues so that the universe doesn't do it for us.

—

The only things that stop healing from happening are fear, doubt, disbelief, and lack of virtues.

—

Start the digging work

Each client you interact with is a stepping-stone to soul ascension. Every new client gives you the opportunity to develop virtues. While every client can teach us something new about the digging process – which can then be used with others – it is also important to understand what it teaches you about yourself and your beliefs. While the process shouldn't be about you, it is still useful to energy test for similar beliefs *after the session* that can then be shared with the client.

Virtue Exercise

Pair up with another person and take turns sharing what is going on in your life and what you have learned from these life experiences.

With each experience, talk about what virtue you have gained from it and the virtues that your soul would like to develop.

Then take turns in the role of practitioner and energy test to see if the other person (in the role of the client) has received the learning so they can move beyond that lesson.

THE DANCE

The final step in belief work is to put all these 10 digging methods together so they become a beautiful dance; a healing art that benefits not only the client but also you. No one should feel tortured in a belief-work session. When the client leaves, they should be radiating joy and knowledge. If you are working on yourself, you should be excited to work on yourself. If you know how to put all the different digging approaches into one session, the client will feel secure. And by continuing to do belief work on yourself, you will become a more accomplished and effective healer.

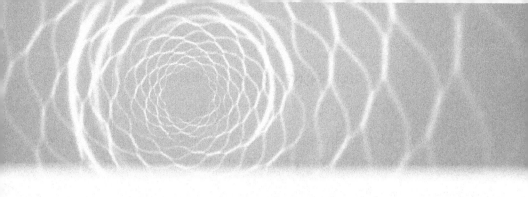

CONCLUSION: BEING A THETAHEALER

Remember what it means to be a ThetaHealer:

A ThetaHealer works with others to discover limiting beliefs that keep them from what they want.

A ThetaHealer teaches others how to embrace their beliefs.

A ThetaHealer teaches others how to ask the Creator for help.

A ThetaHealer teaches others how to become divine beings.

A ThetaHealer teaches others that it is good to go to the doctor.

A ThetaHealer teaches others it is OK to go to a healer.

A ThetaHealer teaches others it is OK to see a spirit, that they are not crazy, and how to send it to the light.

—

**We teach people how to live and
become who they really are.**

—

Here follow some downloads:

'I know what it feels like to put the interests of my client above my own.'

'I know how to co-create with the Creator.'

'I know how to dig for the key belief from a Seventh-Plane perspective.'

'I know how to use all the methods of the digging work in a session.'

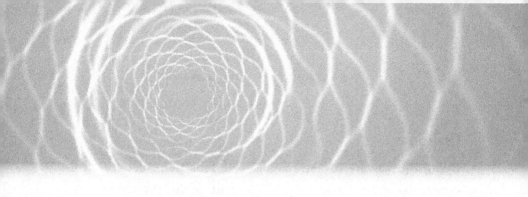

GLOSSARY

Belief system

An individual's or social group's set of beliefs about what is right and wrong and what is true and false.

Belief work

A process of pulling and replacing belief systems.

Body language

Physical movements that express an individual's emotions and state of mind.

Chain of beliefs

Beliefs that are stacked on top of one another, which make up a belief system. *See also* **belief system**.

Conscious

Being fully aware of actions and self. It is theorized that the conscious mind only runs 10 percent of the brain and the subconscious the remaining 90 percent. *See also* **subconscious**.

Core beliefs

One of the four levels of belief. Behavior patterns in the subconscious mind from this life – and mostly stemming from childhood – which have become a part of our programs. Often, this is an effort on the part of the subconscious to protect us and keep us safe. When working on this level the practitioner will witness changes in the frontal lobe. *See also* **four levels of belief**, **programs**, and **subconscious**.

The Creator of All That Is

The most intelligent, perfect love energy in which everything in existence is created.

Crystal layout

A technique to retrieve genetic and past-life memories.

Digging work

A process to find a chain of beliefs that are stacked on top of one another and to change the bottom or key belief. *See also* **chain of beliefs.**

Divine timing

Knowing your destiny and allowing the universe to come in and help you.

Downloads

A process of witnessing positive affirmations coming down from the Creator of All That Is into the mind as though it were a computer. *See also* **Creator of All That Is**.

Energy testing

A process in Thetahealing to test for belief systems. *See also* **belief system**.

Feeling work

A process to teach feelings from the Creator's perspective. For example: God's perspective of virtues such as kindness, patience, non-judgment, etc. *See also* **Creator of All That Is**.

Four levels of belief

There four different levels of belief: core beliefs, genetic beliefs, history beliefs, and soul beliefs. *See also* **core beliefs, genetic beliefs, history beliefs,** and **soul beliefs**.

Free will

Free will is the ability to choose what you believe. It is a Law of the universe that can't be broken.

Gene work

A process to positively influence the structure of a gene karma. There are three types of karma:

- Karma of now.

- Karma of genetics.

- Karma of past lives.

The karma of now are things done in the present that create karma. For example, if you treat someone badly, they treat you badly in return. The karma of genetics means an inherited trait from an ancestor, as well as the karma associated with them. The karma of past lives is bringing karma forward from a past life. These are ancient Hindu beliefs, but in modern times this is known more familiarly as cause and effect.

Genetic beliefs

One of the four levels of belief. Beliefs we have inherited from our parents and ancestors, up to seven generations forward and seven generations back. *See also* **four levels of belief** and **seven generations forward and seven generations back.**

Healing system

A process of co-creating while in a Theta state in order to witness the Creator doing a healing. Helping the body to heal and recover. *See also* **Creator of All That Is** and **Theta state.**

History beliefs

One of the four levels of belief. These beliefs are from past-life memories, and there are many reasons for them, including:

- Behavior patterns from more than seven generations in the past.

- Energies from the Akashic records.

- Collective consciousness memories from personal past-life experiences.

The past-life energy of others is left as imprints from past experiences embedded in inanimate objects. In every grain of sand there are memories of everything that has ever lived on the Earth – experiences that we carry into the present from many lives. *See also* **four levels of belief**.

Manifesting

Imagining what you want and creating it.

Oath (or vow)

A solemn promise or assertion. A declaration that may have been made in another time or place or one made by an ancestor that may or may not serve someone in the present.

Planes of Existence

In ThetaHealing the term is used to describe the seven different planes or realms which are separated by the movement of atoms:

- First Plane: atoms come together moving slowly to form solids, e.g. minerals.

- Second Plane: atoms begin to move faster to form plants.

- Third Plane: realm of animals and proteins.

- Fourth Plane: spirit realm.

- Fifth Plane: realm of the ascended masters.

- Sixth Plane: the Laws of the universe.

- Seventh Plane: an All That Is energy that moves in all things. The beginning and the end.

Programs

Behavior patterns that have been created by beliefs in the mind.

Reading

When a ThetaHealer does a body scan on another person to get imprints of what is happening to them physically, emotionally, mentally, spiritually and in their future.

Release work

Releasing old emotions or programs. *See also* **programs**.

Seven generations forward and seven generations back

Genetic beliefs that are changed on a genetic level and also changed seven generations forward and seven backward in the genetic line. *See also* **genetic beliefs**.

Seventh Plane of Existence

The pure energy of creation which folds into our universe and creates quarks which create protons, neutrons, and electrons which create atoms which create molecules.

Sleep cycle

A time period of usually eight hours in which deep Theta and Delta states of sleep anchor new knowledge in the brain.

Soul beliefs

One of the four levels of belief. These are the deepest and most pervasive of all the belief programs. If a belief is repeated on more than one level, it can go all the way to the soul level. Even though your soul is from God, it is always learning. *See also* **four levels of belief**.

Subconscious

The part of the mind that runs the autonomic systems of the body, as well as some feelings and memories. Its main objective is to keep us safe and alive. The mental activity just below the threshold of consciousness. *See also* **conscious**.

Theta brainwave

A dreamlike state in which brainwaves slow down to between four and seven cycles per second.

Theta state or Theta brainwave state

A very deep state of relaxation; a creative, inspirational state characterized by spiritual sensations.

Ultimate truths

A truth that is absolute such as the sun will rise, the Earth will turn, or a dog is a dog.

Vow

See Oath.

REFERENCES

1. Jha, A. 2005. 'Where belief is born.' Available at: www. theguardian.com/science/2005/jun/30/psychology. neuroscience; accessed January 21, 2019

2. '10 Huge Benefits of Theta Binaural Beats.' Available at: www.binauralbeatsfreak.com/brainwave-entrainment/ the-benefits-of-theta-binaural-beats; accessed January 21, 2019

3. Birney, E. 2015. 'Study of Holocaust survivors finds trauma passed on to children's genes.' Available at: www.theguardian .com/science/2015/aug/21/study-of-holocaust-survivors-finds- trauma-passed-on-to-childrens-genes; accessed January 21, 2019

4. Hughes, V. 2013. 'Mice Inherit Specific Memories, Because Epigenetics?' Available at www.nationalgeographic.com /science/phenomena/2013/12/01/mice-inherit-specific- memories-because-epigenetics/; accessed January 21, 2019

5. Gabbatiss, J. 2018. 'Interstitium: New organ discovered in human body after it was previously missed by scientists.' Available at: www.independent.co.uk/news/health/new-organ- human-body-interstitium-cancer-skin-scientists-discovery-new- york-a8275851.html; accessed January 30, 2019

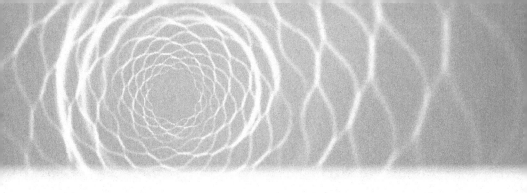

RESOURCES

ThetaHealing Seminars

ThetaHealing is an energy-healing modality founded by Vianna Stibal, with certified instructors around the world. The seminars and books of ThetaHealing are designed as a therapeutic self-help guide to develop the ability of the mind to heal. ThetaHealing includes the following seminars and books:

ThetaHealing® seminars taught by certified ThetaHealing® instructors

ThetaHealing Basic DNA 1 and 2 Practitioner Seminar

ThetaHealing Advanced DNA 2½ Practitioner Seminar

ThetaHealing Manifesting and Abundance Practitioner Seminar

ThetaHealing Intuitive Anatomy Practitioner Seminar

ThetaHealing Rainbow Children Practitioner Seminar

ThetaHealing Disease and Disorders Practitioner Seminar

ThetaHealing World Relations Practitioner Seminar

ThetaHealing DNA 3 Practitioner Seminar

ThetaHealing Animal Practitioner Seminar

ThetaHealing Dig Deeper Practitioner Seminar

ThetaHealing Plant Practitioner Seminar

ThetaHealing SoulMate Practitioner Seminar

ThetaHealing Rhythm Practitioner Seminar

ThetaHealing Planes of Existence Practitioner Seminar

ThetaHealing Growing Your Relationship Instructor Classes

ThetaHealing You and Your Significant Other Seminar

ThetaHealing You and the Creator Seminar

ThetaHealing You and Your Inner Circle Seminar

ThetaHealing You and the Earth Seminar

Certification seminars taught exclusively by Vianna at the ThetaHealing® Institute of Knowledge

ThetaHealing Basic DNA 1 and 2 Instructors' Seminar

ThetaHealing Advanced DNA 2½ Instructors' Seminar

ThetaHealing Manifesting and Abundance Instructors' Seminar

ThetaHealing Intuitive Anatomy Instructors' Seminar

ThetaHealing Rainbow Children Instructors' Seminar

ThetaHealing Disease and Disorders Instructors' Seminar

ThetaHealing World Relations Instructors' Seminar

ThetaHealing DNA 3 Instructors' Seminar

ThetaHealing Animal Instructors' Seminar

ThetaHealing Dig Deeper Instructors' Seminar

ThetaHealing Plant Instructors' Seminar

ThetaHealing SoulMate Instructors' Seminar

ThetaHealing Rhythm Instructors' Seminar

ThetaHealing Planes of Existence Instructors' Seminar

ThetaHealing Growing Your Relationship Certification Classes

ThetaHealing You and Your Significant Other Instructors' Seminar

ThetaHealing You and the Creator Instructors' Seminar

ThetaHealing You and Your Inner Circle Instructors' Seminar

ThetaHealing You and the Earth Instructors' Seminar

ThetaHealing is always growing and expanding, and new courses are added often. Please visit www.thetahealing.com for latest updates.

Books

ThetaHealing® (Hay House, 2006, 2010)

Advanced ThetaHealing® (Hay House, 2011)

ThetaHealing® Diseases and Disorders (Hay House, 2012)

On the Wings of Prayer (Hay House, 2012)

ThetaHealing® Rhythm for Finding Your Perfect Weight (Hay House, 2013)

Seven Planes of Existence (Hay House, 2016)

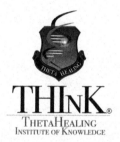

THETAHEALING INSTITUTE OF KNOWLEDGE®
ATANAHA
29048 BROKEN LEG ROAD, BIGFORK, MONTANA 59911
USA

OFFICE: (406) 206 3232
E-MAIL: INFO@THETAHEALING.COM
WEB: WWW.THETAHEALING.COM

ABOUT THE AUTHOR

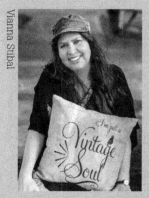

Vianna Stibal

Vianna Stibal is the creator and founder of the spiritual philosophy, meditation, and healing technique known as ThetaHealing®. A renowned healer, author, and motivational speaker, Vianna conducts seminars with her husband, Guy, all over the world to people of all races, beliefs, and religions. As of 2019, she had trained thousands of instructors and an estimated 600,000 practitioners who are working in over 180 countries.

Vianna's technique takes the mind to a deep theta state (dream state) instantaneously. Using this state, she teaches her students to reestablish their conscious connection with the Creator of All That Is to facilitate spiritual, mental, emotional, and physical changes.

After witnessing her own healing, Vianna discovered how emotions and beliefs affect us on core, genetic, history, and soul levels. From this breakthrough, was born the belief work that became the heart and soul of ThetaHealing.

Belief work is a guide to find what we believe, why we believe, and how to change beliefs, change illness, understand the Creator's true plan, and create the reality we desire.

Vianna teaches that we are sparks of God creating our own reality, and that everything in our life serves a purpose. She is dedicated to sharing her love for the Creator of All That Is with an honest humor and a genuine kindness. Her trainings and books are life changing and continue to help people all over the world.

www.thetahealing.com

HAY HOUSE
Online Video Courses

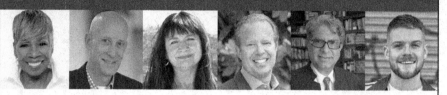

Your journey to a better life starts with figuring out which path is best for you. Hay House Online Courses provide guidance in mental and physical health, personal finance, telling your unique story, and so much more!

LEARN HOW TO:

- choose your words and actions wisely so you can tap into life's magic

- clear the energy in yourself and your environments for improved clarity, peace, and joy

- forgive, visualize, and trust in order to create a life of authenticity and abundance

- manifest lifelong health by improving nutrition, reducing stress, improving sleep, and more

- create your own unique angelic communication toolkit to help you to receive clear messages for yourself and others

- use the creative power of the quantum realm to create health and well-being

To find the guide for your journey,
visit www.HayHouseU.com.

HAYHOUSE
online learning

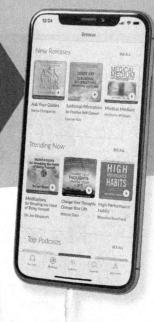

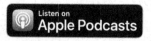

HAY HOUSE
Look within

Join the conversation about latest products, events, exclusive offers and more.

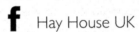 Hay House UK

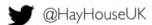 @HayHouseUK

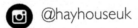 @hayhouseuk

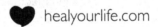 healyourlife.com

We'd love to hear from you!